Medical Nutrition Therapy Simulations

SeAnne Safaii-Waite, PhD, RDN, LD

Associate Professor
University of Idaho
Boise, Idaho

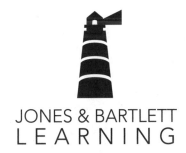

JONES & BARTLETT
LEARNING

World Headquarters
Jones & Bartlett Learning
5 Wall Street
Burlington, MA 01803
978-443-5000
info@jblearning.com
www.jblearning.com

Jones & Bartlett Learning books and products are available through most bookstores and online booksellers. To contact Jones & Bartlett Learning directly, call 800-832-0034, fax 978-443-8000, or visit our website, www.jblearning.com.

Substantial discounts on bulk quantities of Jones & Bartlett Learning publications are available to corporations, professional associations, and other qualified organizations. For details and specific discount information, contact the special sales department at Jones & Bartlett Learning via the above contact information or send an email to specialsales@jblearning.com.

Copyright © 2019 by Jones & Bartlett Learning, LLC, an Ascend Learning Company

All rights reserved. No part of the material protected by this copyright may be reproduced or utilized in any form, electronic or mechanical, including photocopying, recording, or by any information storage and retrieval system, without written permission from the copyright owner.

The content, statements, views, and opinions herein are the sole expression of the respective authors and not that of Jones & Bartlett Learning, LLC. Reference herein to any specific commercial product, process, or service by trade name, trademark, manufacturer, or otherwise does not constitute or imply its endorsement or recommendation by Jones & Bartlett Learning, LLC and such reference shall not be used for advertising or product endorsement purposes. All trademarks displayed are the trademarks of the parties noted herein. *Medical Nutrition Therapy Simulations* is an independent publication and has not been authorized, sponsored, or otherwise approved by the owners of the trademarks or service marks referenced in this product.

There may be images in this book that feature models; these models do not necessarily endorse, represent, or participate in the activities represented in the images. Any screenshots in this product are for educational and instructive purposes only. Any individuals and scenarios featured in the case studies throughout this product may be real or fictitious, but are used for instructional purposes only.

16108-3

Production Credits

VP, Executive Publisher: David D. Cella
Publisher: Cathy L. Esperti
Acquisitions Editor: Sean Fabery
Associate Editor: Taylor Maurice
Director of Vendor Management: Amy Rose
Vendor Manager: Molly Hogue
Director of Marketing: Andrea DeFronzo
VP, Manufacturing and Inventory Control: Therese Connell

Composition: SourceHOV LLC
Project Management: SourceHOV LLC
Rights & Media Specialist: Thais Miller
Media Development Editor: Shannon Sheehan
Cover Image: ©Mazzur/ShutterStock, Inc.
Printing and Binding: Edwards Brothers Malloy
Cover Printing: Edwards Brothers Malloy

Library of Congress Cataloging-in-Publication Data

Names: Safaii-Waite, SeAnne, author.
Title: Medical nutrition therapy simulations / SeAnne Safaii-Waite.
Description: Burlington, MA : Jones & Bartlett Learning, [2019] | Includes
    bibliographical references.
Identifiers: LCCN 2017038373 | ISBN 978-1-284-16107-6 (pbk.: alk. paper)
Subjects: | MESH: Nutrition Therapy | Nutrition Assessment | Nutritionists–education | Simulation Training
Classification: LCC RM216 | NLM WB 18.2 | DDC 615.8/54–dc23
LC record available at https://lccn.loc.gov/20170383736048

6048

Printed in the United States of America
21 20 19 18 17   10 9 8 7 6 5 4 3 2 1

*This book is dedicated to the memory of
Dr. Samantha Ramsay. Her passion for dietetics
lives on in those she touched.*

–SeAnne Safaii-Waite

Contents

Preface

Preparing dietetic students for practice demands that academic and practice-based educators use transformative strategies to develop clinical reasoning skills. Simulation has been increasingly adopted as a teaching methodology in healthcare professions. Dietetic simulation is valued for its ability to provide realistic, context-rich experiential learning in a safe environment. From standardized patients, to low- and high-fidelity mannequins, or virtual patients using decision trees, each context provides a unique perspective and can facilitate the learning and evaluation of patient care situations along the continuum of care.

Medical Nutrition Therapy Simulations guides students through clinical experiences where they practice critical thinking skills. This toolkit is designed to enhance learning content delivered in classroom lectures with activities based on "visiting" the patients in the hospital, providing a perfect environment for students to practice what they learn. By immersing students in a realistic yet safe, clinical environment, students get acclimated to the routine and rigors of the average clinical rotation where they can:

- Conduct a complete nutrition assessment of a patient
- Collect, analyze, and interpret data
- Set priorities for nutrition care plans
- Document conclusions about complex problems

Each lesson should be accompanied by a reading assignment, completion of the decision-tree module available online, and then simulation activities based on "visiting" the patients in the hospital. The toolkit provides a perfect environment to practice and prepare for clinical rotations.

▶ The Contents

The toolkit includes the following components:

Chapter 1: Introduction to Dietetic Simulation

This chapter introduces the teaching method of clinical simulations. Simulation is defined and explained through theory and pedagogy. The debriefing and evaluation process is thoroughly explained so that students understand the expectations of the methodology.

Chapter 2: Nutrition Assessment

This chapter introduces the process of nutrition screening and assessment, and the dietitian's role in preventing malnutrition and improving patient outcomes. Components of each are outlined to prepare students for their decision tree exercises and simulation scenarios.

Simulation Scenarios

The simulation scenarios included in this text are documents outlining the various details of a simulation. Each simulation includes the following sections:

- *Learning Objectives* establishing the measurable outcomes

- *Student and Instructor Preparation* outlining what students and instructors should do prior to initiating the simulation
- *Lab Set Up* describing the patient's characteristics, environment, needed lab staff, and equipment
- *Clinical Case Information* presenting the results of the objective and subjective evaluation, medication orders, progress notes, and lab results
- *Resources* indicating where students and instructors can find additional information
- *Key Words* highlighting terminology with which the student should be familiar

This text includes 10 simulations in total, covering the following topics:

- Celiac disease
- Congestive heart failure
- Chronic obstructive pulmonary disease
- Type 1 diabetes mellitus
- Type 2 diabetes mellitus
- Liver disease
- Lung cancer
- Pancreatitis
- Renal failure
- Wound care

The simulation scenarios are nonsequential and can be taught in any order.

Online Decision-tree Modules

Each new copy of this text includes access to 10 decision-tree modules focused on the same topics as the in-text simulation scenarios. Decision trees are a teaching method in which choices or outcomes of treatment are uncertain and are determined by choices that the student makes. In medical nutrition therapy decision making, there are many situations in which decisions must be made effectively and reliably. The 10 decision trees in this resource are designed as conceptual, simple, decision-making models with the possibility of automatic learning. Like the in-text simulation scenarios, the decision-tree modules are nonsequential and can be used in any order.

▶ How to Use This Product

Ideally, students will complete the decision-tree module for each topic prior to their clinical simulation experience for that condition. This will help them prepare for the simulation scenarios. The decision trees help students collect information, make decisions, and set priorities in a digital manner without direct interaction with their patient. They are given immediate and direct feedback upon completion. The decision trees may be used for practice, or the instructor may incorporate them into the student performance evaluation. Each decision tree has the functionality of automatic grading as pass or fail.

The ten simulation scenarios found in this text have been designed for use in a number of settings, including hospitals, clinics, classrooms, and simulation labs. The simulations can be used with high- or low-fidelity simulation robots or in role-play activities with preceptors or with actors.

▶ Instructor Resources

In order to assist instructors with the 10 simulation scenarios found in this text, an Instructor Manual is available with the following components for each scenario:

- Actor roles and behavior overview
- Scenario events and expected actions
- Debriefing points
- ACEND Competencies
- ADIME note example
- Simulation evaluation instrument

Acknowledgments

I would like to acknowledge and express my sincere thanks to all of those who have contributed to this publication. To Rebekah Ramsey for her incredibly creative and clinical mind in helping develop our simulation scenarios, and to Sue Linja for her expertise, patience, and faith in this project. To the following preceptors and instructors who pilot tested our scenarios: Barbara Gordon, Michon Williams, Courtney Tucker, Teresa Thaut, Krista Brown, Cassi Watkins, Emily Bartell, Ashley Eachon, Cassandra Partridge; Le Greta Hudson and Jennifer Bean from the University of Missouri; and Brooke Schantz Fosco from Dominican University. To my University of Idaho colleagues Sonya Meyer, Hydee Becker, Katie Brown, Katie Miner and Martha Raidl.

A big thank you to all of the dietetic educators who participated in the needs assessment and focus groups that laid the groundwork for the content and format for the simulation scenarios and decision trees.

I would like to thank the amazing team at Jones & Bartlett Learning, including Sean Fabery who spent countless hours putting the format of this resource into place. To the many others who have helped and supported this resource behind the scenes, you do exemplary work, and I salute you!

And last but not least, a big thank you to my husband John and our children who have provided support and encouragement in the balance between family and profession.

About the Author

SeAnne Safaii-Waite, PhD, RDN, LD is an Associate Professor of Nutrition and Dietetics at the University of Idaho. She is a nutrition communications professional, a registered dietitian researcher, and an educator.

SeAnne has been using simulation learning techniques in her medical nutrition therapy and clinical classes for the last 6 years. Her research interests are in simulation and self-efficacy, virtual worlds, diabetes, and aging. She is currently conducting research on aging and diet, specifically as it relates to centenarians from around the world. Her work has been featured in the *Food & Nutrition* magazine, *Today's Dietitian*, and Diabetescare.net. She loves sharing nutrition information in the media, writes for three newspapers, makes appearances on local television networks, tweets, blogs, has given a TEDx talk, and runs an informational website called thecentenariandiet.com. The author of many journal articles, book chapters and a co-author of the newly released book *The Alzheimer's Prevention Food Guide*, she has been the recipient of the Academy of Nutrition and Dietetics' Young Dietitian of the Year Award, the Outstanding Dietitian Award, and most recently the University of Idaho Community Outreach and Engagement Award.

An important aspect of SeAnne's life is family: her husband, daughters, and sons. Together they lead a very active lifestyle cycling, running, skiing, and just about anything that gets them outdoors. One of her favorite foods is pizza, and she hopes to see her 100th birthday!

CHAPTER 1

Introduction to Dietetic Simulation

LEARNING OBJECTIVES

- Define simulation
- Outline the five-component framework for a simulation model
- Understand the value of debriefing
- Identify the MNT Evaluation Score Sheet Components

▶ What Is Simulation?

Clinical simulations are the newest technologic innovation to enter the clinical education environment. Clinical simulation embodies advanced technology and a new way of thinking about education. In postsecondary healthcare fields and continuing education for healthcare professionals, clinical simulation is increasingly recognized as a teaching resource to reduce pressure on the limited access to hospitals and clinics. Simulation is defined by Levett-Jones and Lapkin (2014) as "a technique used to replace or amplify real experiences with guided experiences that evoke or replace substantial aspects of the real world in a fully interactive manner." The confidence of students who have used simulation is increased, patient safety is improved, and rigor is added to the credentialing and precepting process. Simulation reveals similarities to rehearsals in other fields.

During the past decade, real life clinical simulations have been used successfully in healthcare education to train medical and nursing students (Aronson, Rosa, Anifinson, & Light, 1997). A meta-analysis was completed by McGaghie and colleagues (2011) comparing simulation-based medical education with deliberate practice. Their findings revealed that clinical skills acquired in medical simulation laboratory settings transfer directly to improved patient care and better patient outcomes. Unfortunately, most dietetics clinical simulations have relied on either paper case study simulations or role playing and have not advanced to using high-fidelity computerized patients. As a result, dietetic students have limited experience with many clinical conditions. They can often feel overwhelmed and unprepared when they begin their supervised clinical practice. Additionally, accessibility to clinical sites has become increasingly difficult and competitive, and supervised practice/internship requirements have increased. It is to overcome these barriers that this resource, which includes ten clinical dietetics simulations, was developed. Upon completion of these simulations, it is anticipated that students will: (1) acquire clinical reasoning skills that are needed when students are providing Medical Nutrition Therapy (MNP); (2) feel more confident and competent during their clinical supervised practice; (3) be rated by their preceptors as having better clinical reasoning skills; and (4) improve self-efficacy.

▶ Advantages of Simulation

Simulations provide the following advantages:

- This technology can provide realistic clinical experiences without risk to patients and learners. Essentially, learners have "permission to fail" and learn from such failure in a way that would be unlikely in a clinical setting.
- Students can be exposed to clinical experiences that they would rarely see because events can be scripted and practiced. This is important for those interns who may wind up in rural or specialty hospitals or for online learners.
- Scenarios can be designed with comorbidities, increasing complexity, and introduced in a controlled way.
- Skills can be practiced repeatedly, tested, and tailored to individual needs.
- Simulation-based learning can help students to bridge the gap between classroom and clinical settings and support their ability to apply what they have learned.
- Learning is interactive and includes immediate feedback.

- Sessions can be videotaped for subsequent review and discussion, fostering reflective learning, and connecting classrooms in several geographic locations.
- Several learners can benefit from a session and they can learn from each other's successes and mistakes.

In most dietetic-supervised practice experiences, "hands on" dietetic education is provided to students by having them first "see one" of their preceptors demonstrate clinical skills with a patient, after which they have the opportunity to "practice" their own clinical skills with that or another patient. Students are not born with clinical reasoning skills; the skills are learned and developed with time, training, practice, and repetition, which is provided by simulations.

Simulations can also improve faculty, student, and preceptor productivity. Faculty can use simulations for teaching and providing immediate feedback. Students can increase their level of productivity by learning new skills in simulation scenarios before entering the hospital environment. These staged simulation activities will give the students an opportunity to think critically and solve problems in a safe environment. Preceptor productivity would be improved since the simulation would teach the students introductory clinical reasoning skills for ten disease entities. Having learned these skills before entering the hospital, students can progress at a faster pace and be able to work with more patients.

The current method of training dietetics students in a clinical setting, which includes observation and repetition, has shortcomings. The student is in the clinical setting for a short period of time and is exposed to a limited number of cases based on "time and chance." Simulation could mitigate this inherent variability in training, ensuring that all students gain experience with many types of medical conditions—either real or simulated. A new paradigm is required to meet the conflicting demands of the exponentially growing field of dietetics and the ever-decreasing contact time that interns get with individual patients. Dietetic interns who make a mistake in real patient care will never forget it—and likely never repeat it. However, this is helpful only for the *next* patient. Simulation promises to provide such instructive encounters in an artificial environment; yet, it is transferrable to the clinical setting, thereby accelerating the development of expertise while minimizing patient risk.

A two-part, five-component framework for designing simulated dietetics experiences is used in this resource. Each simulation has an accompanying digital decision tree that the students may first practice on their own or in a computer lab to check their MNT skills for that specific disease entity. Next, they complete the simulation scenario, which is composed of five elements. First, each of the simulation scenarios begins with measurable learning objectives. Second, the simulations emulate reality and are based on authentic cases. Third, the simulations move from simple tasks, such as anthropometric measures, to more advanced and complex issues involving higher levels of uncertainty. Fourth, each scenario includes cues from the patient that may include verbalizations, laboratory values, comments from nurses' notes, physician orders, etc., which help students prioritize problems (Aronson et al., 1997). Fifth, the debriefing process, which includes a systematic review, positive and negative feedback, along with suggestions for improvement, is critical to simulation. Debriefing provided after a simulation is the single most important element of the learning experience (Gibbons et al., 2002; Jeffries, 2012; McGaghie, Issenberg, Petrusa, & Scalese, 2006; Thompson & Gutschall, 2005).

▶ The Learning Theory Behind Simulation

Theoretical Basis for Simulation is commonly used in fields characterized by complex, highly technical environments in which conditions change frequently, crises can occur rapidly, and

human life may be at risk. Examples include the aerospace industry, the military, and the nuclear power industry. Several theories are relevant to the use of simulation in education. Waldner and Olson (2007) combine Benner's (1984) *novice-to-expert model* and Kolb's (1984) theory of *experiential learning* to explain how clinical simulation experiences can be used to bring nursing students to higher levels of expertise in nursing practice. Students are expected to progress to at least the advanced beginner level of expertise by graduation. The process of reflecting on clinical practice experiences and theoretical knowledge learned in the classroom is ongoing and continues after graduation as new graduates gain competence and eventually transform into highly competent professionals.

Kolb (1984) describes how active reflection is used by students to incorporate new experiences into their existing skillset and achieve higher levels of expertise in their fields. Students accommodate and assimilate benefit from active experimentation in combination with active reflection to help internalize knowledge. Students may want to experiment with different responses, some of which may be incorrect, in order to learn what would happen and why certain responses are contraindicated in some emergencies. Such experimentation would be unthinkable in an actual clinical setting but could provide a valuable learning experience in a virtual reality setting where there is no risk of patient injury (Sewchuck, 2005).

Teachers are essential to the success of using learning activities, such as simulation. In traditional classroom settings, instruction is teacher-centered, whereas simulation is student-centered, with the teacher playing the role of the facilitator in the student's learning process. In the teaching or facilitating context, the teacher provides learner support, as needed, throughout the simulation and the debriefing that concludes the experience. Teachers may require initial training or video-assisted training on how to use simulation effectively in order to feel comfortable with the experience.

Students must be self-directed and motivated during the simulation, which is more likely to happen if they know the ground rules for the activity. Competition during a simulation experience can be a human motivator. If the simulation involves role-playing, the instructor should inform students about the specific roles they are to play, particularly if the students are to work in groups. Roles vary with the case scenario. For example, one student may play the patient, another may play the family member, and another may play the dietitian. Students should rotate through assigned roles and talk about the various roles during debriefing. Progress toward attaining designated learning outcomes is judged during student evaluations.

Educational Practices involve pedagogic principles that, if used correctly, achieve student learning. These principles include *active learning*, where students are learning through activities that involve the activity and immediate feedback. Case scenarios can be tailored by the instructor to match the skill level of the student—simple to complex. For example, if the student is competent in basic nutrition counseling, the preceptor may adlib more challenging feedback from the patient. Such active and interactive learning environments engage students in the learning process and encourage them to make connections between and among concepts. Simulation experiences can take on the role of individual education plans, tailored to the student's strengths or weaknesses. This is more difficult to do in the traditional classroom or clinic (Ericsson, 2004; Sewchuck, 2005).

Immediate *feedback* is a critical component to help students learn and practice concepts about how their performance, knowledge, and decision-making skills meet the desired learning outcomes. Informed feedback can be useful to build on students' existing knowledge and to help them gain confidence. Cycles of learning are greatly enhanced in simulation with near-instant feedback.

Student-faculty interaction involves discussion about lecture content and how this applies to the scenario. Aronson and colleagues (1997) recommend that faculty members should remain with one clinical scenario during 2 days of teaching for consistency. Faculty is then available to the students to ask questions when completing their nutrition care process notes.

According to Gibbons and colleagues (2002), *collaborative learning* during simulations increases a sense of collegiality and teamwork, which results in faculty–student bonding. Collaborative learning involves sharing different ideas in a group, bringing course content to life without the stress of a real patient, and increasing confidence by giving opportunities for critical thinking and decision-making within their groups. This is another advantage over traditional models.

A teacher's *expectations* for the student to do well tend to become a self-fulfilling prophecy. It is important for students to set goals with the faculty and seek advice on how to achieve those goals. When both faculty and students have high expectations for the simulation process and its outcomes, positive results can be achieved. Vandrey and Whitman (2001) asserted that students can be pushed to expand their competency levels and become empowered to achieve greater learning in a safe environment using simulations where the instructor feels free to intervene and demonstrate the best practice instantly.

Using simulation helps meet the diverse learning styles of students. Dietetics programs often have both traditional college-age students and nontraditional adult learners in the same classroom setting. This increasing diversity of the student population has implications for faculty as they develop their teaching strategies, curriculum, and program development. Simulations can accommodate diverse learning styles and teaching methods and allow students and groups with varying cultural backgrounds to benefit from the experience. For example, the simulation patient can have limited English-speaking ability. A student can be challenged on his or her cultural sensitivities and ability to communicate in these settings.

Outcomes typically associated with undergraduate dietetics include knowledge, skills, student satisfaction, critical thinking, self-efficacy, and meeting competencies. Fuszard (1995) has shown that didactic knowledge gained from simulations is retained longer than knowledge gained through lectures. Simulation experiences also allow for the use of checklists as measures of skill competencies. Both qualitative and quantitative methods can be used to measure students' responses to the experience. Several studies used the Facione California Critical Thinking Skills Tests (CCTST) to assess the critical thinking abilities of students. Additionally, video vignettes have been used to enhance students' critical thinking ability in nursing programs (Chau et al., 2001). Another indicator of student success is *self-efficacy*. At least one university dietetics program has studied the positive effects of classroom simulation on the self-efficacy related to medical nutrition therapy among dietetics students (Parker & Myrick, 2010; Safaii & Ramsay, 2011).

▶ The Pedagogy

A variety of learning theories was used in the development of these medical nutrition therapy scenarios and decision trees. These include, but are not limited to, the following.

Transformative Learning Theory suggests that experiences, either real or simulated, are simple catalysts for learning. Simulation takes knowledge gained from MNT lectures and advances learning by simulating medical scenarios in a safe environment where students are free to make mistakes. The learning does not take place until after the experience, that is, during the debriefing. Comprehensive

student growth and success will result from student engagement in the scenarios. Research indicates that the more engaged the learner is, the bigger the chances of his or her success in the module. Students with high self-efficacy have higher engagement (Fencl & Scheel, 2005; Parker & Myrick, 2010).

The learning *theory of deliberative practice* is also applicable to virtual reality clinical simulations. This set of instructional principles has been demonstrated by instructional science research to be effective in helping students gain expertise in clinical medicine, aviation, *professional sports*, musical performance, and other fields. The principles relate the development of proficiency to the student's engagement in the deliberate practice of desired outcome goals. Outcomes are accomplished by repeated performance of desired cognitive and/or *psychomotor* skills, along with rigorous assessments that give the student specific feedback and facilitate improved skills performance.

Successful learning from the use of simulations requires proper simulation design and evaluation. The simulation model in **FIGURE 1.1** has five major components with associated variables. The outcomes presented in the framework are proposed to be influenced by the degree to which best practices in education are incorporated in the design and implementation of the simulations. Effective teaching and learning using simulations are dependent on teacher and student interactions, expectations, and roles of each during these experiences (Ericsson, 2004; Kolb, 1984; Sewchuck, 2005).

▶ Transformative Teaching

In the simulations, the learner is allowed to discover what they already know, believe, and can do. Whole-person learning requires

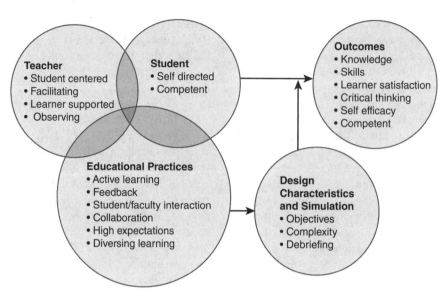

FIGURE 1.1 Simulation model.

that critical reflection and affective learning are integrated into the main learning experience and this will be demonstrated in the debriefing sessions of each simulation. For real transformation to occur, there is a need for learning to take place in a safe, open, trusting environment, which is exactly what simulation fosters (Fencl & Scheel, 2005).

▶ What Is Debriefing?

Adults learn best when they are actively engaged in the process and can bring in their own experiences as a learner. Simulation stimulates both the cognitive and emotional learning. The learner makes sense of the events experienced in their own world. Debriefing sessions should be tailored to the learning objectives, the scenario, and the experience of the participant. Although each scenario comes with its own set of objectives, some may emerge and evolve with the simulation. For example, the objective for a scenario with a patient with COPD may be to identify different nutrition interventions for that patient given his or her

living environment and resources. During the course of the simulation, the student may observe that the patient is uninterested in changing his or her diet. That, in turn, elicits the student's response to turn to motivational interviewing techniques to determine what areas of the diet that patient may be willing to change. Although the objective of this scenario is not to assess the student's skills at motivational interviewing, this objective may emerge as a result of the encounter.

The debriefing session provides students with the opportunity to examine their performance against the goals. Not only do instructors/preceptors share their assessment with the student but students may also be asked to reflect on the emergent objectives and to assess how the behaviors, attitudes, and choices uncovered in the simulation relate to real-life situations. To debrief about such objectives is complicated because there are fewer predefined ideas about how the students should have acted. Therefore, the discussion must focus around issues that arise from the events themselves and their meaning to those involved in the simulation (Anderson, 2008).

▶ The Role of the Debriefing Facilitator

The purpose of debriefing is to give participants time to reflect; discuss the simulation experience; and analyze, synthesize, and evaluate their actions. Students discuss what happened during the simulation, why certain actions were chosen, and what they learned from it. Participants also discover and address any changes needed to improve their patient outcomes (Jeffries, 2012). The debriefing facilitator may be an instructor, preceptor, or a person who is directly involved in the student learning process.

The role of the debriefing facilitator is very important. If he or she uses a judgmental approach, it can have a negative effect on students, such as humiliation, confusion, and decreased motivation and involvement. The facilitator guides the conversation without lecturing and clarifies by providing constructive feedback and active listening techniques are promoted. The facilitator should identify pertinent elements of the simulation and relate these to the objectives.

It is ideal to debrief in a quiet room that is separate from the active simulation area. The room should be comfortable, private, and intimate. The timing of the debriefing is crucial and should occur immediately after the simulation so that thoughts, feelings, and actions are not forgotten. There are many models for debriefing and each debriefing session should last long enough to ask the students the following questions:

- Reactions phase
  - What were your first impressions of the scenario?
  - Was the patient presenting symptoms that you expected?
  - How do you feel it went?

- Analysis phase
  - Did you have the knowledge and skills to meet the objectives?
  - In what ways was the scenario challenging?
  - What went well?
  - What could have been changed?

- Summary phase
  - What was the rationale for what was done and the interventions?
  - Which three factors were significant enough for you to transfer to the clinical setting?
  - In real life, what might you do differently in the future?
  - Is there anything else you would like to discuss?

Sample debriefing questions are outlined as part of the instructor resources for each scenario of this toolkit.

▶ Evaluating Student Performance

Each competency area of clinical nutrition is measured using the MNT Simulation Evaluation Instrument. A pass/fail criterion is used, meaning that the student demonstrates or does not demonstrate competency. To pass the simulation, students need to receive a minimum of 75% on the rubric. Students who do not score 75% will need to repeat the simulation until they score 75%. The score sheet is adaptable to the number of areas under each ADIME criterion that is used. For students who earn between 75% and 85%, it is highly recommended that they write out a self-study action plan on how they will learn the skills needed within the simulation.

Using a combination of lecture, digital decision trees, and simulation can be important educational strategies to prepare students for the real clinical world. **FIGURE 1.2** summarizes the flow of how these enhancement resources can be used.

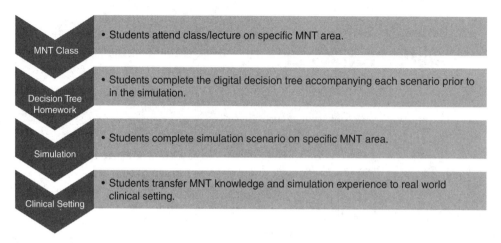

FIGURE 1.2 Transformative teaching.

▶ Supplemental Resources

The scenarios were designed for use in a variety of settings—hospitals, institutions, clinics, classrooms, or simulation labs. The simulations can be used with high- or low-fidelity simulation robots, in role-play activities with preceptors, or with actors. Each scenario will make reference to the Academy of Nutrition and Dietetics Evidence Based Library, Nutrition Care Manual, and ACEND Competencies. These are three critical ancillaries (Accreditation Council for Education in Nutrition and Dietetics, 2016).

MNT SIMULATION COMPONENTS

Both instructors and students see the following components of each simulation:

Learning Objectives – This section outlines the measurable objectives.

Lab Set Up – This section describes what is necessary to set the scene for the scenario.

Student and Instructor Preparation – This section covers reading material necessary for students to complete the scenario.

Clinical Case Information – This section contains information from the patient's medical record needed for students to make decisions regarding the patient's nutrition care.

Instructors also have access to the following items:

Simulation Scenario for Instructors – This section is for instructors only. It guides the instructors/preceptors/actors through each scenario and includes timeframe, patient actions, and expectations from students and cues for patients to use.

Scenario Events and Expected Actions – This section is for instructors only. It is a guided tool for instructors to use for expected actions from the students.

Debriefing Points – This section includes a standardized set of debriefing questions to be used by the instructor with individual students after each scenario or with groups of students, if they are completing simulation in groups.

ACEND Competencies – The Accreditation Council for Education in Nutrition and Dietetics accreditation and competency standards identified for each scenario.

ADIME Note – This section includes sample assessment, diagnosis, intervention, monitoring, and evaluation notes for each scenario.

MNT Simulation Evaluation Instrument – This is an optional evaluation instrument against which to measure student performance. Because it is competency based, students will either meet the competency (1 point) or not meet it (0 points).

▶ References

Accreditation Council for Education in Nutrition and Dietetics. (2016). *ACEND Accreditation Standards for Nutrition and Dietetics*. Available from www.eatright.org/ACEND

Anderson, M. (2008). *Debriefing and guided reflection*. Available from http://www.sirc.nln.org (accessed September 2016).

Aronson, B. S., Rosa, J. M., Anifinson, J., & Light, N. (1997). Teaching tools. A simulated clinical problem-solving experience. *Nurse Educator, 22*(6), 17–19.

Benner, P. (1984). *From novice to expert: Excellence and power in clinical nursing practice*. Menlo Park, CA: Addison-Wesley.

Chau, J., Chang, A., Lee I., Ip, W., Lee, D., & Wootton, Y. (2001). Effects of using videotaped vignettes on enhancing students' critical thinking ability in a baccalaureate nursing program. *Journal of Advanced Nursing, 36*, 112–119.

Ericsson, K. (2004). Deliberate practice and the acquisition and maintenance of expert performance in medicine and related domains. *Academic Medicine, 79*(10, Suppl.), S70–S81.

Fencl, H., & Scheel, K. (2005). Research and teaching: Engaging students—An examination of the effects of teaching strategies on self-efficacy and course in a nonmajors physics course. *Journal of College Science Teaching, 35*(1), 20–24.

Fuszard, R. (1995). *Innovative teaching strategies in nursing* (2nd ed.). Gaithersburg, MD: Aspen Publishers.

Gibbons, S., Adamo, G., Padden, D., Ricciardi, R., Graziano, M., Levine, E., & Hawkins, R. (2002). Clinical evaluation in advanced practice nursing education: Using standardized patients in health assessment. *Journal of Nursing Education, 41*, 215–221.

Jeffries, P. R. (2012). A framework for designing, implementing and evaluating simulations used as teaching strategies in nursing. *Nursing Educator Perspectives, 86*(6), 706–711.

Kolb, D. (1984). *Experiential learning: Experience as the source of learning and development*. Englewood Cliffs, NJ: Prentice Hall.

Levett-Jones, T., & Lapkin, S. (2014). A systematic review of the effectiveness of simulation debriefing in health professional education. *Nurse Education Today, 34*(6), 58–63.

McGaghie, W. C., Issenberd, B., Cohen, J., Barsuk, H., & Wayne, D. (2011). Does simulation-based medical education with deliberate practice yield better results than traditional clinical education? A meta-analytic comparative review of the evidence. *Academic Medicine, 86*, 706–711.

McGaghie, W. C., Issenberg, S. B., Petrusa, E. R., & Scalese, R. J. (2006). Effect of practice on standardized learning outcomes in simulation based medical education. *Medical Education, 40*(8), 792–797.

Parker, B., & Myrick, F. (2010). Transformative learning as a context for human patient simulation. *Journal of Nursing Education, 49*(6), 326–332.

Safaii, S., & Ramsay, S. (2011, September). The effect of classroom simulation on dietetics students' self-efficacy related to medical nutrition therapy. *American Dietetic Association Annual Conference*.

Sewchuck, D. (2005). Experiential learning: A theoretical framework for perioperative education. *AORN Journal, 81*(6), 1311–1318.

Thompson, K., & Gutschall, M. (2005). The time is now: A blueprint for simulation in dietetics education. *JAND, 115*(2), 169–324.

Vandrey, C., & Whitman, M. (2001). Simulator training for novice critical care nurses. *American Journal of Nursing, 101*(9), 24GG–24LL.

Waldner, M. H., & Olson, K. H. (2007). Taking the patient to the classroom: Applying theoretical frameworks to simulation in nursing education. *International Journal of Nursing Education Scholarship, 4*(1), Article 18.

CHAPTER 2

Nutrition Assessment

LEARNING OBJECTIVES

- Define the consequences of malnutrition in hospitalized patients
- Explain the difference between nutrition screening and nutrition assessment
- Identify the components involved in nutrition assessment
- Describe components of the nutrition-focused physical assessment that contributes to the nutrition diagnosis of malnutrition

▶ Malnutrition

Malnutrition is a debilitating and prevalent condition in hospital settings that may affect as many as 30% to 50% of patients, depending on the screening tools used. Often, a patient's nutritional status can deteriorate during his or her hospital stay (American Society for Parenteral and Enteral Nutrition [A.S.P.E.N.], 2013; Barker, Gout, & Crowe, 2011; Fessler, 2008). Malnutrition can lead to poor wound healing, higher rates of infection, greater length of stay, and increased hospital costs. Early nutritional screening and assessment can lead to interventions that can prevent the onset of malnutrition and its related complications and thereby decrease the cost of care (Correia & Waitzberg, 2003; White et al., 2012).

There are many causes of hospital malnutrition. These include failure to track accurately height, weight, and weight loss; failure to observe food intake; skipping or withholding meals due to tests; increased needs due to injury or illness; and delayed nutritional support. Consequently, nutrition screening, assessment, and intervention are critical for the identification of patients who are either malnourished or are at risk for malnutrition (Tappenden et al., 2013; White et al., 2012).

Nutrition screening has been defined by the American Society for Parenteral and Enteral Nutrition (A.S.P.E.N.) as "a process to identify an individual who is malnourished or who is at risk for malnutrition to determine if a detailed nutrition assessment is indicated" (A.S.P.E.N., 2010). In a 2012 consensus statement, the Academy of Nutrition and Dietetics (the Academy) and A.S.P.E.N. defined malnutrition as the presence of two or more of the following characteristics (White et al., 2012):

- Insufficient energy intake
- Weight loss

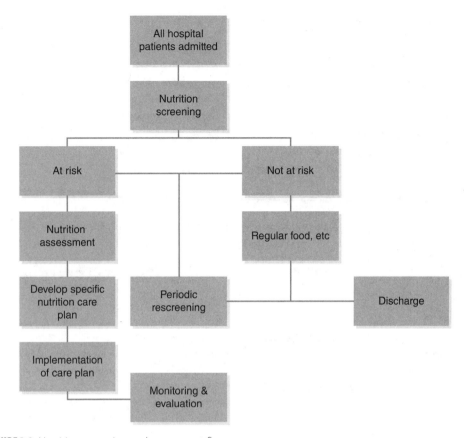

FIGURE 2.1 Nutrition screening and assessment flow.

- Loss of muscle mass
- Loss of subcutaneous fat
- Localized or generalized fluid accumulation
- Decreased functional status

The last four of these characteristics are best assessed by a physical examination (see "Clinical Examination—Nutrition-Focused Physical Exam" in this chapter). Sometimes, observing the muscle or fat loss might be more insightful of a patient's nutritional status than completing a simple diet recall.

Nutrition assessment is conducted on those who are identified as "at risk" and the assessment provides further investigation of these risks (Joint Commission on Accreditation of Healthcare Organizations [JCAHO], 2017). Nutrition assessment has been defined by A.S.P.E.N. as "a comprehensive approach to diagnosing nutrition problems that uses a combination of the following: medical, nutrition, and medication histories; physical examination; anthropometric measurements; and laboratory data." The nutrition assessment provides the foundation for the nutrition intervention.

FIGURE 2.1 demonstrates the nutrition screening and assessment process (Ukleja et al., 2010).

▶ Nutrition Screening

Nutrition screening is a first-line, quickly performed process, which is conducted by a qualified healthcare professional within 24 hours of admission. It identifies those patients who are malnourished or at nutrition risk (Rasmussen, Holst, & Kondrup, 2010). The Joint Commission for Accreditation of Health Care Organizations (JCAHO) recommends nutritional screening within 24 hours of hospital admission with a full nutrition assessment for patients found to be "at risk" (JCAHO, 2017; Nagel, 1993).

Through the identification of nutritional risk, the probability of a better or worse outcome due to nutritional factors can be determined. Each institution will have its own recommended nutrition screening tool and protocol. However, in general, nutrition screening includes reviewing the following risk criteria:

1. Unintentional weight change-illness—**TABLE 2.1** can be used to determine malnutrition criteria for unintended weight loss (Acevedo, 2011; Tappenden et al., 2013).
2. Nutrition History
   a. Reduced food intake (<50% of normal for 5 days)
   b. Appetite
   c. Nausea/vomiting (>3 days)

TABLE 2.1 Unintended Weight Loss Criteria for Malnutrition

Loss of Total Body Weight	Length of Time
More than 2%	In 1 week
More than 5%	In 1 month
More than 7.5%	In 3 months
More than 10%	In 6 months
More than 20%	In 1 year

Reproduced from White J., et al. (2012). Consensus Statement: Academy of Nutrition and Dietetics and American Society for Parenteral and Enteral Nutrition. *Journal of Parenteral and Enteral Nutrition, 36*(3), 275–283.

   d. Diarrhea
   e. Dysphagia
3. Feeding modality
   a. TPN/PPN
   b. TF
   c. Dietary Restrictions
4. Diagnosis—GI symptoms, wounds, cachexia, end-stage liver or kidney disease, coma, malnutrition, decubitus ulcers, cancer, Crohn's Disease, Cystic Fibrosis, new onset diabetes, eating disorders.
5. Laboratory data related to blood proteins.

▶ Nutrition Assessment

Once a patient has been identified to be "at risk" through the screening process, a nutrition assessment is completed. The first step of any assessment is to establish rapport and trust with the patient. The purpose of the nutrition assessment is to obtain, confirm, and interpret data needed to identify nutrition-related problems, their causes, and the significance to the patient's prognosis. To do this, the patient must feel comfortable discussing health concerns and the clinician must be an empathic listener. Nutrition assessment is ongoing and includes continual analysis of the patient's status and the monitoring and evaluation of their progression. The components of nutrition assessment are outlined below (Litchford, 2012; Tappenden et al., 2013).

Medical and Social History

The medical and social history is gathered from the electronic medical record of patient chart and from the patient interview. Medical data include obtaining an individual's medical and surgical history, which includes any diseases or illnesses, prior diagnostic procedures or current treatments and medications, alcohol and drug use, and bowel habits. Some diseases or treatment procedures may increase specific nutrient needs or contribute to malabsorption, which increases the risk of developing a nutritional deficiency. It is also important to determine whether an individual is taking any vitamins, minerals, or herbal supplements, which can affect nutritional status.

Psychosocial data include economic status, marital status, occupation, education level, living and cooking arrangements, mental status, age, sex, level of physical activity, and social support network.

Diet History and Intake

Diet history and intake is gathered from the patient interview. The interviewer should review the patient's appetite, nausea, vomiting, diarrhea, constipation, difficulty in swallowing, food intolerance or preferences, mouth sores, and food intake prior to and after being admitted. The interviewer should also consider factors such as taste changes, dentition, dysphagia, feeding independence, and vitamin/mineral supplements. Estimating the typical caloric and nutrient intake using a 24-hour recall, food-frequency questionnaire, food diary, or observation is also necessary for the purpose of comparing with estimation of caloric needs. Additionally, the interviewer should review typical eating patterns such as daily and weekend diet restrictions, ethnicity, eating away from home, fad diets, and cultural or religious restrictions.

IDEAL BODY WEIGHT CALCULATION (HAMMWI METHOD)

Males: 106 lbs + 6 lbs per inch over 5 ft
Females: 100 lbs + 5 lbs per inch over 5 ft
Add 10% for large frames and subtract 10% for small frames

%IBW = (current wt/IBW) × 100
80–90% mild malnutrition
70–79% moderate malnutrition
60–69% severe malnutrition

Anthropometrics

Assessment of the patient's weight is another critical component of the nutrition assessment. It is important to review the patient's height, usual weight, current weight, weight changes in the last 1 and 5 years prior to being admitted. The patient should also be assessed for edema and/or abnormal swelling.

▶ Biochemical Data

Components of nutritional status can be assessed through laboratory testing or biochemical data. Biochemical data may be obtained through blood, urine, and stool samples. Hydration level, underlying medical conditions, and metabolic processes, like extreme stress, can affect the outcome of biochemical data; therefore, it is important to consider laboratory results as a part of a whole.

For example, hemoglobin and ferritin blood tests reflect iron status; inflammation can be assessed with albumin and C-reactive protein blood levels; cholesterol and lipoprotein blood test results indicate heart disease risk; analyzing stool samples may uncover the presence of blood, indicative of abnormal gastrointestinal tract bleeding; urine sample analysis can provide information on diabetes risk and can alert both patient and healthcare provider to early signs of deteriorating kidney function when high protein levels are present.

By comparing laboratory results with standard values, the determination of any abnormalities can be assessed. Biochemical data can also include drug nutrient interactions. For example, warfarin is an antagonist of vitamin K, making blood clot more slowly, so it is important for patients on warfarin to ingest consistent levels of vitamin K every day.

For additional laboratory assays for vitamin and minerals status, one may refer to *The Nutrition Focused Physical Exam Pocket Guide* published by the Academy (Mordarski & Wolff, 2015).

▶ Clinical Examination— Nutrition-Focused Physical Exam

A nutrition-focused physical exam (NFPE) is a focused, systematic head-to-toe assessment of a patient's physical appearance and function to help determine nutritional status by uncovering any signs of malnutrition, nutrient deficiencies, or nutrient toxicities (Dennett, 2016; Litchford, 2012, 2013; Mordarski & Wolff, 2015).

The NFPE should begin by requesting permission from the patient or his or her family. The patient should be examined visually to identify physical signs of nutrition status. Start from the top; a patient with protein-calorie malnutrition may have dry, easily pluckable or sparse hair; skin may be pale and dry; dehydration may be seen in poor skin turgor; poor wound healing may be linked to deficiencies of protein, vitamin C, and zinc. Areas of concern that may be identified as signs of malnutrition are included in **TABLE 2.2**.

TABLE 2.2 Physical Exam: Parameters Useful in the Assessment of Nutritional Status

Exam Areas	Tips	Severe Malnutrition	Mild-Moderate Malnutrition	Well Nourished
Subcutaneous fat loss				
Orbital Region – Surrounding the Eye	View patient when standing directly in front of them, touch above cheekbone	Hollow look, depressions, dark circles, loose skin	Slightly dark circles, somewhat hollow look	Slightly bulged fat pads. Fluid retention may mask loss
Upper Arm Region – Triceps/biceps	Arm bent, roll skin between fingers, do not include muscle in pinch	Very little space between folds, fingers touch	Some depth pinch, but not ample	Ample fat tissue obvious between folds of skin
Thoracic and Lumbar Region – Ribs, Lower Back, Midaxillary line	Have patient press hands hard against a solid object	Depression between the ribs very apparent. Iliac Crest very prominent	Ribs apparent, depressions between them less pronounced. Iliac Crest somewhat prominent	Chest is full, ribs do no show. Slight to no protrusion of the iliac crest.
Muscle loss				
Temple Region – Temporalis Muscle	View patient when standing directly in front of them, ask patient to turn head side to side	Hollowing, scooping, depression	Slight depression	Can see/feel well-defined muscle
Clavicle Bone Region – Pectoralis Major, Deltoid, Trapezius Muscles	Look for prominent bone. Make sure patient is not hunched forward	Protruding, prominent bone	Visible in male, some protrusion in female	Not visible in male, visible but not prominent in female

Exam Areas	Tips	Severe Malnutrition	Mild-Moderate Malnutrition	Well Nourished
Clavicle and Acromion Bone Region – Deltoid Muscle	Patient arms at side; observe shape	Shoulder to arm joint looks square. Bones prominent. Acromion protrusion very prominent	Acromion process may slightly protrude	Rounded, curves at arm/shoulder/neck
Scapular Bone Region – Trapezius, Supraspinus, Infraspinus Muscles	Ask patient to extend hands straight out, push against solid object.	Prominent, visible bones, depressions between ribs/scapula or shoulder/spine	Mild depression or bone may show slightly	Bones not prominent, no significant depressions
Dorsal Hand – Interosseous Muscle	Look at thumb side of hand; look at pads of thumb when tip of forefinger touching tip of thumb	Depressed area betweeen thumb-forefinger	Slightly depressed	Muscle bulges, could be flat in some well nourished people
Lower body less sensitive to change				
Patellar Region – Quadricep Muscle	Ask patient to sit with leg propped up, bent at knee	Bones prominent, little sign of muscle around knee	Knee cap less prominent, more rounded	Muscle protrude, bones not prominent
Anterior Thigh Region – Quadriceps Muscles	Ask patient to sit, prop leg up on low furniture. Grasp quads to differentiate amount of muscle tissue from fat tissue.	Depression/line on thigh, obviously thin	Mild depression on inner thigh	Well rounded, well developed
Posterior Calf Region – Gastrocnemius Muscle	Grasp the calf muscle to determine amount of tissue	Thin, minimal to no muscle definition	Not well developed	Well-developed bulb of muscle
Edema				
Rule out other causes of edema, patient at dry weight	View scrotum/vulva in activity restricted patient; ankles in mobile patient	Deep to very deep pitting, depression lasts a short to moderate time (31–60 sec) extremity looks swollen (3–4+)	Mild to moderate pitting, slight swelling of the extremity, indentation subsides quickly (0–30 sec)	No sign of fluid accumulation

Reproduced from Mordarski, B., & Wolff, J. (2015). *Nutrition focused physical exam pocket guide.* Chicago, IL: Academy of Nutrition and Dietetics.

▶ Putting It All Together

Learning the nutrition assessment takes time, clinical experience, and practice. It is better to start small, mastering one or two specific areas of your assessment at a time and build one's skills from there. Components of the nutrition assessment, mentioned in this chapter, are included in most institutional protocols; however, each institution has its own set of unique requirements. The latest addition to the nutrition assessment procedure is nutrition-focused physical assessment. Some institutions have been slower than others at standardizing these procedures into their dietetic practice. Regardless of institutional protocol, ACEND includes a new competency, which requires that students are able to conduct nutrition-focused physical exams.

▶ References

Acevedo, M. G. (2011). *Nutrition assessment: Tools & techniques.* McLean, VA: Nutrition Dimension. Available at: http://www.continuingeducation.com/pdf/rd100_elt-nas-11.pdf

American Society for Parenteral and Enteral Nutrition (A.S.P.E.N.). (2010). American Society for Parenteral & Enteral Nutrition (A.S.P.E.N.) definition of terms, style, and conventions used in A.S.P.E.N. Board of Directors–approved documents. Available at: https://www.nutritioncare.org/WorkArea/DownloadAsset.aspx?id=3613

American Society for Parenteral and Enteral Nutrition (A.S.P.E.N.). (2013). One in three hospitalized patients is malnourished; Experts call for better diagnosis and treatment. Available at: https://www.nutritioncare.org/Press_Room/2013/One_in_Three_Hospitalized_Patients_is_Malnourished;_Experts_Call_for_Better_Diagnosis_and_Treatment/

Barker, L. A., Gout, B. S., & Crowe, T. C. (2011). Hospital malnutrition: Prevalence, identification and impact on patients and the healthcare system. *International Journal of Environmental Research and Public Health, 8*(2), 514–527.

Correia, M. I., & Waitzberg, D. L. (2003). The impact of malnutrition on morbidity, mortality, length of hospital stay and costs evaluated through a multivariate model analysis. *Clinical Nutrition, 22*(3), 235–239.

Dennett, C. (2016). Nutrition-focused physical exams. *Today's Dietitian, 18*(2), 36.

Fessler, T. A. (2008). Malnutrition: A serious concern for hospitalized patient. *Today's Dietitian, 10*(7), 44.

Joint Commission on Accreditation of Healthcare Organizations. (2017). *2017 Comprehensive Accreditation Manual for Hospitals (CAMH).* Chicago, IL: Joint Commission on Accreditation of Healthcare Organizations.

Litchford, M. D. (2012). *Nutrition focused physical assessment: Making clinical connections.* Greensboro, NC: CASE Software and Books.

Litchford, M. D. (2013). Putting the nutrition-focused physical assessment into practice in long-term care. *Annals of Long Term Care, 21*(11), 38–41.

Mordarski, B., & Wolff, J. (2015). *Nutrition focused physical exam pocket guide.* Chicago, IL: Academy of Nutrition and Dietetics.

Nagel, M. (1993). Nutrition screening: Identifying patients at risk for malnutrition. *Nutrition in Clinical Practice, 8*(4), 171–175.

Rasmussen, H. H., Holst, M., & Kondrup, J. (2010). Measuring nutritional risk in hospitals. *Clinical Epidemiology, 2,* 209–216.

Tappenden K. A., Quatrara B., Parkhurst M. L., Malone A. M., Fanjiang. G., & Ziegler, T. R. (2013). Critical role of nutrition in improving quality of care: An interdisciplinary call to action to address adult hospital malnutrition. *Journal of the Academy of Nutrition and Dietetics, 113*(9), 1219–1237.

Ukleja, A., Freeman, K. L., Gilbert, K., Kochevar, M., Kraft, M. D., Russel, M. K., & Shuster, M. H. (2010). Nutrition care algorithm (Adapted from Standards for Nutrition Support: Adult Hospitalized Patients). *Nutrition in Clinical Practice, 25,* 403–414.

White, J. V., Guenter, P., Jensen, G., Malone, A., Schofield, M. (2012). Consensus statement of the Academy of Nutrition and Dietetics/American Society for Parenteral and Enteral Nutrition: Characteristics recommended for the identification and documentation of adult malnutrition (undernutrition). *Journal of the Academy of Nutrition and Dietetics, 112*(5), 730–738.

SIMULATION SCENARIO:

Celiac Disease

LEARNING OBJECTIVES

- Identify the recommended nutrition therapy for celiac disease
- Identify several resources for educating the patient on a gluten-free diet
- Estimate appropriate protein, calorie, and fluid needs for patient based on recommended calculations for estimated needs

▶ Student and Instructor Preparation

- Read chapter and lecture notes on medical nutrition therapy for celiac disease/gluten-free enteropathy
- Understand national MNT guidelines for omitting gluten from the diet, and risk factors including: malnutrition, stress, unhealthy eating habits, smoking, alcohol consumption, family history of gluten intolerance or autoimmune diseases, age, impaired immunity, and chronic disease
- Review Evidence Based Library of the Academy of Nutrition and Dietetics
- Practice online decision-tree module for celiac disease

▶ Lab Set Up

Patient: Brenda Smith

Patient characteristics: Mrs. Smith is a 35-year-old female who is a stay-at-home mom with four children, the youngest of whom is 2 years old. She has a degree in elementary education but is taking time off from work to raise her family. She enjoys running and learning about nutrition and how to cook healthier for her family. She enjoys all kinds of foods and takes her kids to McDonald's once a week for a "treat." She lives close to her in-laws, but she does not get along well with them, so her extended family support is not good. Her family lives in another state, including an older brother and his family, a younger sister and her family, and parents. She tries to limit the stress in her life, but it can be difficult because her husband often works long days as an accountant.

Environment/setting/location: Patient's hospital room, lights on and window curtain open; afternoon visit.

Lab staff needed on day of simulation: Preceptor/evaluator (1) or patient (1) (can be another preceptor/instructor, sim man, another student, or actor) for patient's husband, R.D. in training (or student).

Equipment, supplies, and prop list: Hospital room; privacy curtain hung, separating doorway in patient's room from bed area; patient bed; bedside table; water mug on tray next to bed; chair at bedside. The student dietitian may need to prepare handouts regarding Celiac disease, including menus and recipes that are all gluten free for patient to take home. The dietitian may also need to compile a list of support groups and credible on-line resources that the patient can use from home.

▸ Clinical Case Information (03/08/2017)

Subjective

Mrs. Smith is a 35-year-old female who was admitted to the hospital directly from my office, after a 10-day course of extreme nausea, vomiting, and diarrhea that she reports has been going on for several months but has been getting worse over the past week and a half. Initially, the patient thought she was pregnant, but says she has taken multiple pregnancy tests that have all been negative. She also reports that her periods have become erratic. She says she has tried zofran, and a BRAT diet to reduce nausea and diarrhea but nothing has helped. She has had her thyroid checked, which has come back abnormal and she was started on levothyroxine 75 µg daily about 3 weeks ago. She says she is so tired that she can't get out of bed and she has constant, painful abdominal bloating. She says she just can't eat anything—everything just "goes straight through her." Mrs. Smith has lost 20 lbs in the past 2 months from her UBW of 148 lbs; she now weighs 128 lbs. She says she is having pasty bowel movements that "float" in the toilet, which she has never had in her life except for in the past month. She is worried that she is becoming anemic and malnourished.

Objective
Vital signs

- Blood pressure: 118/79
- Temperature: 98.7°F
- O_2: 97% on room air
- Weight: 128 lbs
- Height: 5'7"
- UBW: 148 lbs

PMHx

Fairly unremarkable except for hypothyroid recently diagnosed. The patient says she is "lactose intolerant."

Past surgical Hx

Right knee surgery in 1997 after a snowmobiling accident, C-section in 2013, LASIK surgery in 2014.

Family Hx

Father with gout and chronic diarrhea of unknown origin. Mother with thyroid disease and elevated cholesterol. Maternal grandmother with macular degeneration, HTN, and DM type 2. Now recalls that she has an aunt on her mother's side with gluten intolerance.

Meds

- Levothyroxine 75 μg daily
- Prenatal vitamin daily
- Vitamin D 2000 IU daily
- Vitamin E 400 μg daily
- She occasionally takes Excedrin Migraine for headaches, but not daily.

Abnormal lab values

- Na^+ 135
- K^+ 3.2 (low)
- Cl 96 (low)
- Osmolality 296
- Gluc 80
- BUN 15
- Cr 0.75
- Albumin 3.2 (low)
- Total protein 6.1 (low)
- Calcium 8.0 (low)
- TSH 4.32
- Hgb 11.8 (low)
- Hct 47.5 (low)
- Normal LFTs, amylase, and lipase values
- Serum iron 22 (low)
- Ferritin 10 (low)
- % Saturation 197 (low)
- TIBC 99 (high)

System review

- Heart: RRR
- Lungs: clear
- Extremities: no edema, cyanosis. Bumpy, itchy rash on patient's mid-back.
- Chest: no rales or wheezing; normal breathing

- CV: unremarkable
- Abdomen: Bloated, tender, and "upset" stomach.
- Neurologic: poor hand-grip strength, otherwise unremarkable.
- Eyes: PERRLA

Assessment/Plan

1. Hyponatremia, hypokalemia—We will initiate NS at 100 mL per hour. We will monitor her electrolytes closely and draw a CMP and CBC daily. Replace electrolytes.
2. GI dysfunction with unknown etiology— We will keep her NPO; we will check for C-diff to r/o toxin; she says the last time she was on an antibiotic was 2 years ago. We will schedule a CT scan of the abdomen to r/o bowel obstruction or ileus. We will initiate oral contrast. We will go ahead and consult Surgery for an endoscopy tomorrow, if bowel obstruction or ileus is negative.
3. Hypothyroidism—She was just started on levothyroxine at 75 μg daily. Will hold oral meds at this time.
4. Abdominal pain—We will offer Dilaudid 0.5 mg IV q 2 to 3 hours for pain.
5. Rash—Mrs. Smith has an itchy, raised rash to her mid-back. She says she has had this on and off for the past 6 months or so. She was going to see a dermatologist but never made the appointment.
6. Iron deficiency anemia—Will follow for results of CT scan.
7. Malnutrition—She certainly fits criteria for severe malnutrition as her intake is reportedly 50% or less of normal intake and she has had a 20-lb weight loss of 13.5% in 2 months.

▶ Medication/Orders

Medication Orders	Amount	Route	Start Date
Levothyroxine	75 μg daily		HOLD
Prenatal vitamins	1 capsule daily		HOLD
Vitamin D-3	2,000 IU daily		HOLD
LR	Initiate at 75 mL/hr Increase to 100 mL/hr within 24 hours	IV	03/08/2017
Electrolyte replacement	15 mL daily	IV	03/08/2017
Dilaudid	0.5 mg q 2 to 3 hrs prn	IV	03/08/2017
CT contrast	360 mL	Oral	03/08/2017

Diet Order

NPO

Therapy Orders

R.D. consult for nutrition prn
S.T. consult prn
Social Services consult prn

▶ Physician Progress Note 03/09/2017

Subjective

The patient reports that her pain has been better with Dilaudid. The CT scan, which was performed on 03/08/2017, reveals dilated small bowel with fluid-filled loops, not uniform in size, with luminal opacification. No bowel obstruction or ileus noted. Findings of CT scan consistent with gluten-sensitive enteropathy, including villous atrophy of small bowel mucosa. Hyponatremia/hypokalemia resolving with IV fluids and electrolyte replacement. The patient is not interested in eating at this point. She remains lethargic and has been sleeping most of the time.

Objective

Vital signs

- Blood pressure: stable at 115/80
- O_2: 95%
- Weight: 128 lbs; no change from weight upon admission

Abnormal lab values

- Hgb 10.3 (low)
- Hct 35.6 (low)

- MCV 78.0 (low)
- MCH 29.8 (low)
- MCHC 29.4 (low)
- Elevated eosinophils
- Total protein 6.2 (low)
- Albumin 3.0 (low)
- Calcium 8.3 (low)
- Positive tTG-IgA antibodies

Meds

Hold all oral meds and continue with IV fluids at 100 mL per hour, as well as IV Dilaudid.

System review

- Heart: RRR
- Lungs: clear
- Extremities: no edema, cyanosis. Bumpy, itchy rash on patient's mid-back.
- Chest: no rales or wheezing; normal breathing
- CV: unremarkable
- Abdomen: Bloated, tender, and "upset" stomach.
- Neurologic: poor hand-grip strength, otherwise unremarkable.
- Eyes: PERRLA

Assessment

1. Hyponatremia/hypokalemia—resolved with IV fluids and electrolyte replacement.
2. GI dysfunction—gluten-sensitive enteropathy. We added a tTG-IgA test to labs today to r/o gluten sensitivity, which was positive. We will conduct an endoscopy today to determine the severity of this disease. The patient will remain NPO until after endoscopy. Anticipate diet advancement to clear liquids by late this afternoon.
3. Pain management—We will continue her on Dilaudid at current rate; patient has been gradually using less for pain management.
4. Rash to mid-back—What resembles dermatitis herpetiformis (DH).

5. Gluten-sensitive markers—tTG-IgA positive. We will probably start the patient on clear liquids later this afternoon and transition to a gluten-free diet as long as she tolerates clear liquids. We will also obtain a dietary consult for gluten-free diet teaching.
6. Iron deficiency anemia—We will go ahead and give the patient a dose of IV iron due to decreased Hgb, decreased Hct, decreased MCV, decreased MCHC, and low serum iron value. We expect that this is largely due to problems #2 and #4.
7. Malnutrition—due to gluten-sensitive enteropathy. With 13.5% weight decline × past 2 months.

▶ Multidisciplinary Progress Notes

Nursing Progress Note 03/08/2017: 1100

Started IV in left hand at 0900; at 1030, the patient pushed the call light and stated that her IV was hurting. R.N. came in to check IV and found that IV had permeated. Discontinued IV in the left hand and was restarted in the right hand. Current IV running at 75 mL per hour and patient tolerating well. Patient is resting in bed with eyes closed. Patient's husband in room at 1045, after new IV started. Procedure was explained to patient's husband and he stated no concerns at this time.

Nursing Progress Note 03/08/2017: 1330

Patient getting ready for CT scan of abdomen at 1345. Vitals done, BP slightly elevated at 120/89, patient reports she is "nervous" but wants to know what is going on so she hopes this works. Reassured patient and told her to try to relax. O$_2$ 94% on room air. Patient trying to rest prior to procedure.

Nursing Progess Note 03/08/2017: 1900

Patient back from CT at 1530; has been resting in bed and asking for physician to come in and explain findings of CT scan. Reassured patient that physician would be in to speak with her as soon as he can. Patient has been pleasant this shift. She is in bed watching T.V. at this time. May benefit from antianxiety medication prn.

Nursing Progress Note 03/09/2017: 0800

Patient up several times through the night to use restroom; otherwise, has slept well. Patient's husband has stayed with her through the night. Patient has no complaints. She is awaiting blood work results today.

Nursing Progress Note 03/09/2017: 1130

Physician in to see patient and discuss results of labs taken today with positive tTG-IgA. Physician ordered a nutrition consult with extensive dietary teaching for a gluten-free diet. Vitals taken. Patient resting in bed.

Nursing Progress Note 03/09/2017: 1400

Patient awaiting dietitian visit to explain dietary implications of gluten-free diet. Patient reports she is a little familiar with foods she should avoid, such as bread, but she reports she is both nervous about this change and relieved to know how she can fix this problem. Patient up to use restroom this afternoon and states she had a loose bowel movement. Continues on IV fluids and Dilaudid.

▶ Labs

CBC—03/08/2017

Test	Result	Units	Reference Ranges
WBC	10.3	×10^3/uL	4.8–10.8
RBC	6.00	×10^3/uL	4.10–6.70
Hemoglobin	11.0 (LO)	g/dL	12.5–16.0
Hematocrit	35.2 (LO)	Percent	37.0–47.0
Erythrocyte MCV	80.0 (LO)	fL	81.0–96.0
Erythrocyte MCH	32.2 (LO)	pg	33.0–39.0

Test	Result	Units	Reference Ranges
Erythrocyte MCHC	30.0 (LO)	g/dL	32.0–36.0
RDW	16.2	Percent	13.0–18.0
MPV	7.9	fL	6.9–10.6
Platelet count	410 (HI)	×10³/uL	130–400
Neutrophils (pct)	40.0	Percent	39.3–73.7
Neutrophils (ct)	2.0	×10³/uL	1.5–6.6
Lymphocytes (pct)	35.4	Percent	18.0–48.3
Lymphocytes (ct)	1.9	×10³/uL	1.1–2.9
Monocytes (pct)	7.8	Percent	4.4–12.7
Monocytes (ct)	0.5	×10³/uL	0.2–0.8
Eosinophils (pct)	8.2 (HI)	Percent	0.6–7.3
Eosinophils (ct)	0.6 (HI)	×10³/uL	0.0–0.4
Basophils (pct)	0.0	Percent	0.0–1.7
Basophils (ct)	0.0	×10³/uL	0.0–0.1

CMP—03/08/2017

Test	Result	Units	Reference Ranges
Sodium	135 (LO)	mmol/L	137–145
Potassium–serum	3.2 (LO)	mmol/L	3.6–5.2
Chloride	96 (LO)	mmol/L	100–110
Glucose	80	mg/dL	60–100

(continues)

Test	Result	Units	Reference Ranges
BUN	15	mg/dL	7–17
Creatinine	0.75	mg/dL	0.52–1.04
Urea nitrogen/Cr ratio	20	Ratio	
GFR	>90	mL/minute	
Osmolality	296		
Uric acid	5.5	mg/dL	2.5–6.2
Total protein	6.1 (LO)	g/dL	6.5–8.1
Albumin	3.2 (LO)	g/dL	3.2–4.4
Globulin	2.89	g/dL	2.7–4.3
Albumin/globulin ratio	1.10	Ratio	
Calcium	8.0 (LO)	mg/dL	8.4–10.2
Bilirubin	0.5	mg/dL	0.2–1.3
ALT	36	U/L	9–52
AST	24	U/L	14–36
Alkaline phosphatase	45	U/L	38–126
Amylase	55	U/L	23–85
Lipase	78	U/L	0–160
Serum iron	22 (LO)	µg/dL	30–170
Ferritin	10 (LO)	ng/mL	12–150
% Saturation	197 (LO)	mg/dL	200–350
TIBC	99 (HI)	µmol/L	45–85

CBC—03/09/2017

Test	Result	Units	Reference Ranges
WBC	10.0	×10³/uL	4.8–10.8
RBC	5.29	×10³/uL	4.10–6.70
Hemoglobin	10.3 (LO)	g/dL	12.5–16.0
Hematocrit	35.6 (LO)	Percent	37.0–47.0
Erythrocyte MCV	78.0 (LO)	fL	81.0–96.0
Erythrocyte MCH	29.8 (LO)	pg	33.0–39.0
Erythrocyte MCHC	29.4 (LO)	g/dL	32.0–36.0
RDW	15.7	Percent	13.0–18.0
MPV	9.2	fL	6.9–10.6
Platelet count	430 (HI)	×10³/uL	130–400
Neutrophils (pct)	46.8	Percent	39.3–73.7
Neutrophils (ct)	4.2	×10³/uL	1.5–6.6
Lymphocytes (pct)	66.2	Percent	18.0–48.3
Lymphocytes (ct)	2.3	×10³/uL	1.1–2.9
Monocytes (pct)	7.3	Percent	4.4–12.7
Monocytes (ct)	0.6	×10³/uL	0.2–0.8
Eosinophils (pct)	8.9 (HI)	Percent	0.6–7.3
Eosinophils (ct)	0.7 (HI)	×10³/uL	0.0–0.4
Basophils (pct)	0.0	Percent	0.0–1.7
Basophils (ct)	0.0	×10³/uL	0.0–0.1

CMP—03/09/2017

Test	Result	Units	Reference Ranges
Sodium	137	mmol/L	137–145
Potassium–serum	3.6	mmol/L	3.6–5.2
Chloride	101	mmol/L	100–110
Glucose	85	mg/dL	60–100
BUN	12	mg/dL	7–17
Creatinine	0.70	mg/dL	0.52–1.04
Urea nitrogen/ Cr ratio	17.1	Ratio	
GFR	>90	mL/minute	
Uric acid	6.0	mg/dL	2.5–6.2
Total protein	6.2 (LO)	g/dL	6.5–8.1
Albumin	3.0 (LO)	g/dL	3.2–4.4
Globulin	3.2	g/dL	2.7–4.3
Albumin/globulin ratio	0.93	Ratio	
Calcium	8.3 (LO)	mg/dL	8.4–10.2
tTG-IgA	Positive		

▶ Nursing Intake and Output Queries

03/08/2017

Intake				
	0000–0800 hrs	0800–1600 hrs	1600–2400 hrs	24-hour total
IV/FL	N/A	819 mL	818.50 mL	1,637.50 mL
PO	NPO	NPO	NPO	NPO
Total	**0 mL**	**819 mL**	**818.50 mL**	**1,637.50 mL**

Output				
	0000–0800 hrs	0800–1600 hrs	1600–2400 hrs	24-hour total
Urine	200 mL	680 mL	600 mL	1,480 mL
BM			Liquid 200 mL	200 mL
Total	**200 mL**	**680 mL**	**800 mL**	**1,680 mL**

24-hour total fluid balance: −42.50 mL.

03/09/2017

Intake				
	0000–0800 hrs	0800–1600 hrs	1600–2400 hrs	24-hour total
IV/FL	818 mL	718 mL	817.50 mL	2,353.50 mL
PO	NPO	NPO	240 mL	240 mL
Total	**818 mL**	**718 mL**	**1,057.50 mL**	**2,593.50 mL**

Output				
	0000–0800 hrs	0800–1600 hrs	1600–2400 hrs	24-hour total
Urine	620 mL	500 mL	360 mL	1,480 mL
BM		Liquid 220 mL		220 mL
Total	**620 mL**	**720 mL**	**360 mL**	**1,700 mL**

24-hour total fluid balance: 893.50 mL.

Meal Record

	Breakfast	Snack	Lunch	Snack	Dinner	Snack	24-hour Total
03/08/2017	NPO		NPO		NPO		NPO
03/09/2017	NPO		NPO		240 mL		240 mL
03/10/2017	360 mL						

Weight Log

	02/22/2017	02/23/2017	02/24/2017	02/25/2017
Method	Bed Scale	Bed Scale	Bed Scale	
Weight (lbs)	128	128	129	
Weight (kg)	58.1	58.1	58.6	
Height (in)	67			

▶ Resources

Evidenced-based practice guidelines, protocols, or algorithms used in creating the scenario include the following. Students may wish to review these resources in preparation for the simulation scenario.

- Kane and Prelack. *Advanced Medical Nutrition Therapy.* Jones & Bartlett Learning: Burlington, 2018.
- Academy of Nutrition and Dietetics. Evidence Based Practice Guidelines.
- Academy of Nutrition and Dietetics. Nutrition Care Manual.
- Safaii-Waite. *Medical Nutrition Therapy Simulations.* Online module: Celiac disease. Jones & Bartlett Learning: Burlington, 2017.

▶ Key Words

Anemic
Autoimmune disease
Celiac Disease
Endoscopy
Gluten-free
Gluten-sensitive enteropathy
Ileus

SIMULATION SCENARIO:

Congestive Heart Failure

LEARNING OBJECTIVES

- Identify different nutrition interventions for CHF and how to select the appropriate intervention
- Be able to identify the recommended nutrition therapy for patients with CHF
- Estimate protein, calorie, and fluid needs for patient

▶ Student and Instructor Preparation

- Read chapter and lecture notes on medical nutrition therapy for CHF/heart failure
- Understand national MNT guidelines for CHF/heart failure and potential risk factors, including: malnutrition, stress, unhealthy eating habits, smoking, alcohol consumption, diabetes, age, and chronic disease
- Review Evidence Based Library of the Academy of Nutrition and Dietetics
- Review equations for estimation of energy, protein needs, and fluid needs for CHF patient
- Practice online decision-tree module for CHF

▶ Lab Set Up

Patient: Joan Bean

Patient characteristics: Mrs. Bean is an 85-year-old female who has been suffering with CHF for several years. She has had three hospitalizations in the past year alone from complications associated with CHF. She lives with her husband in her home and doesn't like to cook much. She enjoys going out to eat with him, so that she doesn't have to use so much energy to cook. She is very sedentary at home as she lacks the energy to do much there. She is tired of coming to the hospital and is especially tired of her diet while here.

Environment/setting/location: Patient's hospital room.

Lab staff needed on day of simulation: Preceptor/evaluator (1) or patient (1) (can be another preceptor/instructor, sim man, another student, or actor), patient's husband at bedside (1) can be another student or actor, (1) student or actor as patient's nurse at the end of the scenario.

Equipment, supplies, and prop list: Hospital room; curtain draped just inside door as privacy barrier; bed with pillow and blanket; chair at bedside for patient's husband; piece of paper to act as diet information handout; and a flipchart or notebook to act as patient's chart.

▶ Clinical Case Information (01/06/2017)

Subjective

Mrs. Bean is an 85-year-old female who presented to the ER with shortness of breath and hypoxia early this morning. She states that she has been taking her medications as prescribed, except that she forgot to fill her diuretic a week ago and has not been able to make it to the pharmacy due to bad weather. She and her husband have no family around to help them pick up their medications. The patient reports that she has gained 10 lbs in the past week, as her UBW is 115 lbs; she thinks it is due to fluid. She c/o swollen legs and she could not get her shoes on this morning.

Objective

$10(56.8) + 6.25(160.02)$

$568 + 1000 - 425$

$- 161$

952

Vital signs

- Blood pressure: 142/80
- Temperature: 98.5°F
- O_2: 87% on room air, now requiring 2 liters O_2
- Weight: 125 lbs
- Height: 5'3"

Meds

- Lorazepam 1 mg daily
- Lasix 40 mg/day
- Levothyroxine 125 µg daily
- Ca^{++} with vitamin D-2 capsules daily
- Omeprazole 40 mg b.i.d.
- Celexa 20 mg daily KCl
- Prednisone 10 mg daily
- Actonel 35 mg once weekly

Abnormal lab values

- Na$^+$ 125 (low)
- K$^+$ 3.3 (low)
- Cl 93 (low)
- BUN 20 (high)
- Cr 1.05 (high)
- Hgb 11.5 (low)
- Hct 33.2 (low)

System review

- Heart: slight physiologic murmur
- Lungs: clear
- Extremities: 3+ edema to bilateral lower legs.
- Chest: no rales or wheezing
- CV: lower-extremity edema, elevated BP.
- Abdomen: Soft, nontender, active bowel sounds.
- Neurologic: unremarkable

Assessment

1. CHF—Exacerbation with fluid retention resulting in hyponatremia and hypokalemia. The patient will be started on IV Lasix and we will diurese her fairly aggressively.
2. Asthma—Continue with prednisone therapy.
3. Anxiety—Continue with lorazepam at current dose.
4. Depression—Patient reports that she has been doing well with Celexa, so this will remain the same.
5. Hypothyroidism—Will continue with current medication and dose.
6. Osteoporosis—Patient continues on Actonel as well as Calcium with vitamin D.

Plan

We will admit her and start IV Lasix and see if we can't get excess fluid removed from her. We will continue her usual oral medications, with the exception of the p.o. Lasix, and get her up and moving with some assistance. We will limit fluids to 1,800 mL restriction and order a 2 gm Na^+ diet. Anticipate a 1- to 2-night stay.

▶ Medication/Orders

Medication Orders	Amount	Route	Start Date
Lisinopril	20 mg daily	p.o.	01/06/2017
Lorazepam	1 mg daily	p.o.	01/06/2017
Levothyroxine	125 µg daily	p.o.	01/06/2017
Omeprazole	40 mg b.i.d.	p.o.	01/06/2017
Celexa	20 mg daily	p.o.	01/06/2017
Prednisone	10 mg/day	p.o.	01/06/2017
Acetaminophen	325 mg q 6 hrs prn	p.o.	01/06/2017
Ondansetron	4–8 mg q 6 hrs prn	p.o.	01/06/2017
Simethicone	80 mg q 2 hrs prn	p.o.	01/06/2017
Actonel	35 mg q week/Sunday	p.o.	01/06/2017
Lasix	80 mg b.i.d.	IV	01/06/2017
KCl in D5W	10 mEq/hr	IV	01/06/2017

Diet

2 gm Na^+ diet

Therapy Orders

P.T. to ambulate twice daily, work with strengthening and balance.
R.D. to consult for nutrition, diet needs prn, encourage diet compliance.
S.T. consult prn.
Social Services consult with discharge planning for possible ECF placement for rehabilitation.

▶ Physician Progress Note 01/07/2017

Subjective

Patient reports she is feeling better today. She has been diuresed through the night and tolerating her diet, although she is not very happy with being on a sodium-restricted diet—medical professionals believe that this greatly contributes to helping her feel better.

Objective

Vital signs

- Blood pressure: stable at 120/80
- O_2: 89% on 1 L oxygen, improved from 2 L yesterday
- Weight: 120 lbs, down 5 lbs from admission R/T to diuresis.

Abnormal lab values

- Na^+ 136 (low)
- K^+ 3.5 (low)
- Cl 99 (low)
- BUN 20 (high)
- Cr 1.09 (high)
- Calcium 7.9 (low)

Meds

- Lorazepam 1 mg daily
- Lasix 40 mg/day
- Levothyroxine 125 µg daily
- Ca^{++} with vitamin D-2 capsules daily
- Omeprazole 40 mg b.i.d.
- Celexa 20 mg daily
- KCl, prednisone 10 mg daily
- Actonel 35 mg once weekly

Assessment

1. Hyponatremia and hypokalemia—resolving. Continue with KCl at current rate, continue with diuresis, and reduce IV Lasix to 20 mg b.i.d. Hopefully, we can get patient on her oral meds by tomorrow and she can go home.
2. Asthma—controlled.
3. Anxiety—controlled with current medication.
4. Hypothyroid—Seems to be controlled with current levothyroxine dose.
5. Renal Insufficiency, CKD stage 3—Could be R/T Lasix therapy, but patient has had HTN for quite some time. Continue to follow renal labs and GFR.
6. Osteoporosis—Continue with Actonel.
7. Depression—Patient seems to think this is working for her.

Plan

We will finish diuresis and move patient back to her oral medications, hopefully by tomorrow, so that she can go home. Will see if we can't get the nutritionist to encourage her with her diet and teach her what she needs to know at home.

▶ Multidisciplinary Progress Notes

Social Services Consult/Discharge Planning Progress Note 01/06/2017: 0930

Patient and family feel that they are able to manage on their own at home if patient is able to continue same level of functioning she is showing in working with P.T.

Physical Therapy Progress Note 01/06/2017: 1045

Patient ambulating without problems, using walker in hallway. Good progress and strength.

Nursing Progress Note 01/06/2017: 1100

Patient just finished working with P.T.; wants to rest before taking a shower. Took all medications without a problem. Frequency of bathroom visits: 3× this shift. Patient getting ready to order lunch, wants a turkey sandwich with a slice of bacon on it for lunch but encouraged patient not to eat bacon.

Nursing Progress Note 01/06/2017: 1600

Patient just took a shower. IV Lasix still at 40 mg b.i.d., frequently using the restroom and slept poorly through the night last night. Patient says she wants to sleep and not be bothered.

Nursing Progress Note 01/07/2017: 0800

Vitals taken. Patient resting quietly in bed.

▶ Labs

CBC—01/06/2017

Test	Result	Units	Reference Ranges
WBC	7.9	×10³/uL	4.8–10.8
RBC	6.01	×10³/uL	4.10–6.70
Hemoglobin	11.5 (LO)	g/dL	12.5–16.0
Hematocrit	33.2 (LO)	Percent	37.0–47.0
Erythrocyte MCV	82.0	fL	81.0–96.0
Erythrocyte MCH	34.5	pg	33.0–39.0

Test	Result	Units	Reference Ranges
Erythrocyte MCHC	35.8	g/dL	32.0–36.0
RDW	14.8	Percent	13.0–18.0
MPV	6.5	fL	6.9–10.6
Platelet count	250	×10³/uL	130–400
Neutrophils (pct)	45.5	Percent	39.3–73.7
Neutrophils (ct)	3.5	×10³/uL	1.5–6.6
Lymphocytes (pct)	33.5	Percent	18.0–48.3
Lymphocytes (ct)	2.5	×10³/uL	1.1–2.9
Monocytes (pct)	5.2	Percent	4.4–12.7
Monocytes (ct)	0.2	×10³/uL	0.2–0.8
Eosinophils (pct)	2.3	Percent	0.6–7.3
Eosinophils (ct)	0.2	×10³/uL	0.0–0.4
Basophils (pct)	0.5	Percent	0.0–1.7
Basophils (ct)	0.1	×10³/uL	0.0–0.1

CMP—01/06/2017

Test	Result	Units	Reference Ranges
Sodium	125 (LO)	mmol/L	137–145
Potassium–serum	3.3 (LO)	mmol/L	3.6–5.2
Chloride–serum	93 (LO)	mmol/L	100–110
Glucose	87	mg/dL	60–100

(continues)

Test	Result	Units	Reference Ranges
BUN	20 (HI)	mg/dL	7–17
Creatinine	1.05 (HI)	mg/dL	0.52–1.04
Urea nitrogen/Cr ratio	19.0	ratio	
GFR	49	mL/minute	
Uric acid	2.5	mg/dL	2.5–6.2
Total protein	6.5	g/dL	6.5–8.1
Albumin	3.1 (LO)	g/dL	3.2–4.4
Globulin	3.4	g/dL	2.7–4.3
Albumin/globulin ratio	0.91	Ratio	
Calcium	7.4 (LO)	mg/dL	8.4–10.2
Bilirubin	0.6	mg/dL	0.2–1.3
ALT	29	U/L	9–52
AST	36	U/L	14–36
Alkaline phosphatase	120	U/L	38–126
TSH	2.20	uIU/mL	0.32–5.00

BMP—01/07/2017

Test	Result	Units	Reference Ranges
Sodium	136 (LO)	mmol/L	137–145
Potassium–serum	3.5 (LO)	mmol/L	3.6–5.2
Chloride–serum	99 (LO)	mmol/L	100–110

Test	Result	Units	Reference Ranges
Glucose	82	mg/dL	60–100
BUN	21 (HI)	mg/dL	7–17
Creatinine	1.09 (HI)	mg/dL	0.52–1.04
Calcium	7.9 (LO)	mg/dL	8.4–10.2

▶ Nursing Intake and Output Queries

01/06/2017

Intake				
	0000–0800 hrs	0800–1600 hrs	1600–2400 hrs	24-hour total
IV/FL				
PO	400 mL	360 mL	100 mL	860 mL
PO	500 mL	240 mL	200 mL	940 mL
Total	**900 mL**	**600 mL**	**300 mL**	**1,800 mL**

Output				
	0000–0800 hrs	0800–1600 hrs	1600–2400 hrs	24-hour total
Urine	500 mL	1000 mL	800 mL	2,300 mL
Urine	450 mL	600 mL	480 mL	1,530 mL
BM				
Total	**950 mL**	**1,600 mL**	**1,280 mL**	**3,830 mL**

24-hour total fluid balance: −2030 mL.

Meal Record

	Breakfast	Snack	Lunch	Snack	Dinner	Snack	24-hour Total
01/06/2017	50%		75%		75%	50%	66% meals
01/07/2017	75%						

Weight Log

	01/06/2017	01/07/2017	01/08/2017	01/09/2017
Method	Bed Scale	Bed Scale		
Weight (lbs)	125	120		
Weight (kg)	56.8	54.5		
Height (in)	63			

▶ Resources

Evidenced-based practice guidelines, protocols, or algorithms used in creating the scenario include the following. Students may wish to review these resources in preparation for the simulation scenario.

- Kane and Prelack. *Advanced Medical Nutrition Therapy*. Jones & Bartlett Learning: Burlington, 2018.
- Academy of Nutrition and Dietetics. Evidence Based Practice Guidelines.
- Academy of Nutrition and Dietetics. Nutrition Care Manual.
- Academy of Nutrition and Dietetics. Academy of Nutrition and Dietetics Health Informatics Infrastructure (ANDHII). https://www.andhii.org/info/.

- Safaii-Waite. *Medical Nutrition Therapy Simulations*. Online module: Congestive heart failure. Jones & Bartlett Learning: Burlington, 2017.

▶ Key Words

CHF
CKD stage 3
Diuresis
Exacerbation
GFR
Hypokalemia
Hypoxia
Osteoporosis
Prednisone
SOB

10 (50.9) + 6.25 (167.64) -5(76) -161
559 + 1,098 - 380 -161

1,016

٬ω٬

SIMULATION SCENARIO:

Chronic Obstructive Pulmonary Disease (COPD)

LEARNING OBJECTIVES

- Identify different nutrition interventions for COPD and how to select the appropriate intervention
- Be able to identify the recommended nutrition therapy for patients with COPD exacerbation
- Estimate protein, calorie, and fluid needs for patient

▸ Student and Instructor Preparation

- Read chapter and lecture notes on medical nutrition therapy for COPD exacerbation
- Understand national MNT guidelines for this disease and potential risk factors, including: malnutrition, stress, unhealthy eating habits, smoking, and environmental exposures
- Review Evidence Based Library of the Academy of Nutrition and Dietetics
- Review equations for estimation of energy, protein needs, and fluid needs for wound patients
- Practice online decision tree module for chronic obstructive pulmonary disease

▸ Lab Set Up

Patient: Bessie Reynolds

Patient characteristics: Bessie is a 76-year-old female who has had COPD for 13 years as a result of a long history of smoking. She lives at home alone in a retirement community. Her husband died 15 years ago from a MI. Her daughter lives nearby and checks on her daily. Bessie lacks the energy to cook decent meals and often, she buys microwavable meals out of convenience. She has a poor appetite and has lost a considerable amount of weight over the years. She has a difficult time eating because she becomes short of breath. She is depressed and is resistant to change her ways. She has a frail appearance and lack of facial expressions due to decreased energy. She appears much older than she really is.

Environment/setting/location: Patient's hospital room.

Lab staff needed on day of simulation: Preceptor/evaluator (1) or patient (1) (can be another preceptor/instructor, sim man, another student, or actor), patient's daughter at bedside (1) can be another student or actor (dressed in isolation clothing).

Equipment, supplies, and prop list: Hospital room, curtain draped just inside door as privacy barrier; bed with pillow and blanket; chair at bedside for patient's daughter; piece of paper to act as diet information handout; an isolation clothing cart outside of the patient's room with multiple changes of clothing, including isolation gowns, surgical gloves, and masks. Provide a sign on the door indicating that the patient is in isolation. Provide hand sanitizer on isolation clothing cart.

▶ Clinical Case Information (03/28/2017)

Subjective

Bessie is a 76-year-old female with COPD for the past 13 years. She was brought into the ER by her daughter, who reports that her mother had become more short of breath over the past 2 days and has been unable to obtain relief through her normal breathing treatments. She denies having a fever or chills.

She has a history of smoking a pack and a half of cigarettes a day for 50 years. She quit 13 years ago at the time of her diagnosis, so she says, but her daughter reports that Bessie still smokes occasionally. This is concerning, especially since she requires oxygen at home. Bessie has also lost a considerable amount of weight over the years. She says she always used smoking as a way to control her weight, but even since she quit, she has continued to lose weight. She also reports a poor appetite and often skips meals due to shortness of breath. Her normal activity consists of sitting in her chair at home and watching T.V. most of the day. She sends her daughter to do her grocery shopping. Bessie often misses her doctor's appointments and puts them off by rescheduling her appointments. She has not followed up with her doctor for close to a year.

Objective

Vital signs

- Blood pressure: 125/87
- Temperature: 100.2°F
- O_2: 86% on her normal 2 liters of oxygen; she is now on 4 liters and saturation is 92%
- Weight: 112 lbs
- Height: 5'6"
- UBW much of adulthood stated at 142 lbs
- BMI = 18.1, she is 30 lbs fewer than her normal adult weight, but it is unknown how long ago this was. The patient seems to think she has lost 30 lbs in the past 5 to 6 years gradually, due to aging. She does appear to have protruding clavicles, fat, and muscle wasting to temporal and spinal regions. She lacks firmness in her handshake/grip strength.

PMHx

Bipolar disorder, depression, CKD stage 3, constipation, allergic rhinitis, osteoporosis, malnutrition.

Surgical Hx

Wrist surgery (right wrist) in 2001 for which she wears a brace daily, tonsillectomy, and adenoidectomy in 1968 for chronic infections, excision of a benign cyst on outer left thigh in 1985. She has had two basal cell carcinomas removed in 1997 from her right lower leg.

Meds

- Acetaminophen 1,000 mg every 6 hours prn
- Docusate sodium two capsules daily for constipation
- Budesonide 400 μg (two inhalations) twice daily
- Fluticasone one spray in each nostril twice daily
- Aspirin 81 mg daily
- Lasix 40 mg daily
- Lithium 900 mg b.i.d.
- Xopenex inhaler
- Methylprednisolone 20 mg daily
- Fosamax 70 mg once weekly

Abnormal lab values

- WBC 11.7 (high)
- Hgb 11.0 (low)
- Hct 34.1 (low)
- Neutrophils elevated
- Sodium 128 (low)
- K^+ 3.0 (low)
- Cl 90 (low)
- Gluc 110 (high)
- BUN 24 (high)
- Cr 1.50 (high)
- Osmolality 270 (low)
- Uric acid 6.6 (high)
- Total protein 6.0 (low)
- Albumin 2.5 (low)
- Calcium 7.1 (low)
- Serum iron 29 (low)
- Ferritin 10 (low)
- % Saturation 178 (low)
- TIBC 92 (high)

System review

- General: She c/o shortness of breath, cough at times, fatigue, poor appetite. Denies fever but was found febrile.
- HEENT: Denies vision problems, c/o chronic runny nose due to allergies.
- Cardiopulmonary: RRR, has hx of heart attack, edema 3+ to bilateral lower extremities. Diminished crackles in lungs, slight wheeze.
- Gastrointestinal: denies heartburn; no abdominal pain; no gastroparesis, diarrhea, or vomiting.
- Genitourinary: denies bleeding or incontinence.
- Musculoskeletal: lethargic, muscle weakness, no c/o joint pain.
- Neurologic: No dizziness, numbness, or tingling in the hands and feet.
- Allergies: Seasonal allergies/allergic rhinitis; citrus fruits, including strawberries.

Assessment/Plan

1. COPD—Exacerbation with fluid retention. We will start the patient on IV Lasix at 4 mg per hour and hopefully transition to p.o. Lasix tomorrow, depending on how much fluid we get from her. We will continue to have R.T. evaluation and treatment. Oxygen requirements increased to 4 liters this a.m. and her oxygen saturations are 92%.
2. Bronchitis—likely viral. We will go ahead and start her on IV ABX; however, she is noted to be MRSA positive from nasal swab. This will influence our choice of antibiotic therapy. We will initiate 1 gram vancomycin IV over the first hour and then reduce the dose to 1 gram IV q 12 hours.
3. Iron deficiency anemia—Serum iron 29 (low), ferritin 10 (low), % saturation 178 (low), TIBC 92 (high). We will give her some iron replacement parenterally and recheck her Hgb and Hct in the morning.

4. Elevated uric acid values—We will discontinue the aspirin as this may be driving up her uric acid levels. We will continue to monitor uric acid while she is here. We will change her aspirin to clopidogrel, as this may have less of an effect on her uric acid levels.

5. HTN with CKD stage 3—The patient initially told me that her doctor never put her on medication. She was prescribed a low-sodium diet to assist with controlling mild HTN. It is uncertain if she follows this; however, given her history of weight loss and poor intake, sodium intake is probably not excessive at this point.

6. Osteoporosis—She continues on weekly Fosamax dose.

7. Bipolar disorder—She is on lithium tablets extended release—900 mg b.i.d. (q 12 hours), both the patient and her daughter deny any concerns with this.

8. Malnutrition—This is definitely an issue given her poor intake and weight loss. We will see if we can't get her eating and try out some nutrition supplements to see what she likes. We will seek a nutrition consult to assist with this.

9. Depression—The patient's daughter reports that the patient initially agreed to try electroconvulsive therapy but never attended her appointments.

▶ Medication/Orders

Medication Orders	Amount	Route	Start Date
Acetaminophen	1,000 mg q 6 hrs prn	p.o.	03/28/2017
Clopidogrel	75 mg daily	p.o.	03/28/2017
Docusate sodium	1 capsule b.i.d.	p.o.	03/28/2017
Lorazepam	1 mg daily	p.o.	03/28/2017
Levothyroxine	125 µg daily	p.o.	03/28/2017
Lithium	900 mg q 12 hrs	p.o.	03/28/2017
Budesonide	400 µg (2) twice daily	inhalation	03/28/2017
Fluticasone	1 spray each nostril Once daily	inhalation	03/28/2017
Furosemide	4 mg/hr	IV	03/28/2017
Fosamax	70 mg once weekly	p.o.	03/28/2017

Medication Orders	Amount	Route	Start Date
Methylprednisolone	20 mg daily	p.o.	03/28/2017
Vancomycin	1 gm Change to 1 gm Q 12 hrs after first hour	IV	03/28/2017
Venofer	200 mg one time	IV	03/28/2017
Xopenex	1 inhalation prn	inhalation	03/28/2017

Diet

2 gm Na$^+$ diet
1200 mL fluid restriction

Therapy Orders

R.T. to evaluate and treat prn. Breathing treatments q 4 hours as needed.
P.T. to ambulate twice daily, work with strengthening and balance.
R.D. consult for nutrition and diet needs, encourage diet compliance, evaluate for KCAL and protein requirements for weight maintenance.
S.T. consult prn.
Social Services consult with discharge planning for possible ECF placement for rehabilitation.

▶ Physician Progress Note 03/29/2017

Subjective

Bessie reports today that she feels about the same. She says she is in pain, that her chest hurts, and she is starting to cough much more. She is tired and somewhat lethargic. She is not interested in eating this morning. She agreed to try some cranberry juice, but only took a few sips of that. Bessie's daughter, Kathy, explained this morning that her mother has had a poor appetite and chooses to eat puddings, ice cream, or sip on Pepsi throughout the day. She says she purchases her mom's food weekly but lately, she has been buying less and less because it is not being eaten. Apparently, Kathy confronted her mother's neighbor who confessed to purchasing cigarettes for her mother. We may need to contact Social Services to see how we can handle this issue if it does not stop.

Objective
Vital signs

- Blood pressure: 129/86
- O$_2$: 92% on 3 L. oxygen, improved from 4 L yesterday.
- Weight: 109 lbs, down 3 lbs from admission R/T to Diuresis.

Abnormal lab values

- WBC 10.9 (high)
- Hgb 11.9 (low)
- Hct 36.1 (low)
- Neutrophils elevated
- Sodium 134 (low)
- K$^+$ 3.2 (low)
- Cl 98 (low)
- Gluc 121 (high)
- BUN 32 (high)

- Cr 1.24 (high)
- Uric Acid 6.5 (high)
- Total protein 6.2 (low)
- Albumin 2.7 (low)
- Calcium 6.5 (low)

Meds

- IV meds include:
  - Furosemide 4 mg/hr
  - Vancomycin 1 gm q 12 hours

- Oral meds:
  - Acetaminophen
  - Clopidogrel
  - Docusate Sodium
  - Lorazepam
  - Levothyroxine
  - Lithium
  - Fosamax 70 mg weekly
  - Methylprednisolone 20 mg daily

- Inhalations:
  - Budesonide
  - Fluticasone
  - Xopenex

Assessment/Plan

1. COPD—Exacerbation with fluid retention. She has been diuresed over the past 24 hours and has had close to 4 liters out. She is breathing easier and her edema is down to 1 to 2+ bilateral lower extremities. She is on 3 liters of oxygen and saturations are 92% with that. We will continue with IV Lasix throughout most of today to see if we can't get a little more fluid off.
2. Bronchitis—She did have a positive MRSA swab from nares. She is on vancomycin IV 1 gram q 12 hours. We will continue with the IV antibiotic today, and she will remain on isolation precautions.
3. Iron deficiency anemia—Serum iron 29 (low), ferritin 10 (low), % saturation 178 (low), TIBC 92 (high) on 3/28/2017. She received a dose of IV iron yesterday.

We are monitoring her Hgb and Hct for changes—although these may also be affected by her fluid status.

4. Elevated uric acid values—She was started on clopidogrel yesterday. We are monitoring her uric acid values to see if they begin to trend down. For now, she will continue on the clopidogrel.
5. HTN with CKD stage 3—We will continue to provide a low-sodium diet and fluid restriction. She is not eating well, but we probably need to be encouraging of following such a diet. There have been no known problems with her compliance to the fluid restriction during this admission.
6. Osteoporosis—She continues on weekly Fosamax dose.
7. Bipolar disorder—She is on lithium tablets extended release—900 mg b.i.d. (q 12 hours). We will not change this at this time.
8. Malnutrition—She has a history of weight loss. She is still not eating well. Hopefully, as she begins to feel better in the next couple days, her intake will improve.
9. Depression—I spoke with the patient and her daughter concerning her aversion to taking an antidepressant. At this time, she does not think that she needs any medication for depression. We will have a consultation with Social Services regarding this and possibly conduct a depression scale.

▶ **Multidisciplinary Progress Notes**

Social Services Consult/Discharge Planning Progress Note 03/28/2017: 1045

Received consult for social services to provide smoking cessation class for patient. Visited the patient this a.m. who refused smoking cessation information and teaching. She states that she does not smoke any longer and has not smoked for more than 10 years.

Was able to encourage the patient to continue to avoid smoking and provided pamphlets with information and resources to aide with smoking cessation at bedside, but patient continued to tell Social Services that she does not smoke. Patient's daughter caught Social Services after visit and explained that she believes that her mother still smokes occasionally and this is very concerning to her since she is on oxygen 24 hours a day. Patient's daughter says she doesn't know how or where her mother would be getting cigarettes from since she purchases all of her groceries. She thinks her mother's neighbor might be providing them for her. She said she will have a talk with her mother's neighbor.

Physical Therapy Progress Note
03/28/2017: 1100

Patient ambulated in the hallway a short way, but asked to go back to her room because she said she was short of breath. Patient relied on physical therapy for support during ambulation. She is weak and barely has energy to move her walker in front of her. Will try ambulation again later this afternoon.

Nursing Progress Note
03/28/2017: 1130

Patient asking her daughter to get her cups of water from the sink in her bathroom. Explained to patient that she is on an 1,800-mL fluid restriction and that Nursing needs to provide her beverages. Also informed patient's daughter of restriction. Vital signs taken without complaint. Patient states she is tired and wants to take a nap. Patient sleeping at this time.

Nursing Progress Note
03/28/2017: 1400

Patient still sleeping. Woke to nurse checking temperature, which is 99.0. Encouraged the patient to order lunch, but patient said she didn't have the energy to eat and that the food was garbage. She requested pain medication this afternoon, stating that her chest hurt from coughing.

Nursing Progress Note
03/28/2017: 2200

Patient refused to ambulate or work with P.T. this eve. She says she is too tired and they make her work too hard. Breathing is labored, but improved from earlier this a.m.

Nursing Progress Note
03/28/2017: 0900

Patient agreed to take a shower this morning. Vitals taken. Patient declined breakfast but said she would drink Ensure. Patient continues on 1,800 mL fluid restriction. Had 4 liters urine out in the past 24 to 36 hours. She prefers to drink water and is taking some juice at mealtimes.

▶ Labs

CBC—03/28/2017

Test	Result	Units	Reference Ranges
WBC	11.7 (HI)	×10³/uL	4.8–10.8
RBC	6.00	×10³/uL	4.10–6.70
Hemoglobin	11.0 (LO)	g/dL	12.5–16.0
Hematocrit	34.1 (LO)	Percent	37.0–47.0
Erythrocyte MCV	82.0	fL	81.0–96.0
Erythrocyte MCH	34.6	pg	33.0–39.0
Erythrocyte MCHC	35.3	g/dL	32.0–36.0
RDW	15.3	Percent	13.0–18.0
MPV	7.9	fL	6.9–10.6
Platelet count	225	×10³/uL	130–400
Neutrophils (pct)	95.0 (HI)	Percent	39.3–73.7
Neutrophils (ct)	7.8 (HI)	×10³/uL	1.5–6.6
Lymphocytes (pct)	40.2	Percent	18.0–48.3
Lymphocytes (ct)	2.3	×10³/uL	1.1–2.9
Monocytes (pct)	12.9 (HI)	Percent	4.4–12.7
Monocytes (ct)	0.7	×10³/uL	0.2–0.8
Eosinophils (pct)	6.8	Percent	0.6–7.3
Eosinophils (ct)	0.4	×10³/uL	0.0–0.4
Basophils (pct)	0.8	Percent	0.0–1.7
Basophils (ct)	0.1	×10³/uL	0.0–0.1

CMP—03/28/2017

Test	Result	Units	Reference Ranges
Sodium	128 (LO)	mmol/L	137–145
Potassium–serum	3.0 (LO)	mmol/L	3.6–5.2
Chloride	90 (LO)	mmol/L	100–110
Glucose	110 (HI)	mg/dL	60–100
BUN	24 (HI)	mg/dL	7–17
Creatinine	1.50 (HI)	mg/dL	0.52–1.04
Urea nitrogen/Cr ratio	16	Ratio	
GFR	50	mL/minute	
Osmolality	270 (LO)	mosm/kg	275–295
Uric acid	6.6 (HI)	mg/dL	2.5–6.2
Total protein	6.0 (LO)	g/dL	6.5–8.1
Albumin	2.5 (LO)	g/dL	3.2–4.4
Globulin	3.5	g/dL	2.7–4.3
Albumin/globulin ratio	0.71	Ratio	
Calcium	7.1 (LO)	mg/dL	8.4–10.2
Bilirubin	1.0	mg/dL	0.2–1.3
ALT	45	U/L	9–52
AST	25	U/L	14–36
Alkaline phosphatase	100	U/L	38–126
Serum iron	29 (LO)	µg/dL	30–170

(continues)

Test	Result	Units	Reference Ranges
Ferritin	10 (LO)	ng/mL	12–150
% Saturation	178 (LO)	mg/dL	200–350
TIBC	92 (HI)	µmol/L	45–85
Serum folate	40.0	nmol/L	4.5–45.3

CBC—03/29/2017

Test	Result	Units	Reference Ranges
WBC	10.9 (HI)	×10³/uL	4.8–10.8
RBC	4.60	×10³/uL	4.10–6.70
Hemoglobin	11.9 (LO)	g/dL	12.5–16.0
Hematocrit	36.1 (LO)	Percent	37.0–47.0
Erythrocyte MCV	82.0	fL	81.0–96.0
Erythrocyte MCH	34.8	pg	33.0–39.0
Erythrocyte MCHC	35.0	g/dL	32.0–36.0
RDW	15.0	Percent	13.0–18.0
MPV	8.2	fL	6.9–10.6
Platelet count	230	×10³/uL	130–400
Neutrophils (pct)	80.5 (HI)	Percent	39.3–73.7
Neutrophils (ct)	7.30 (HI)	×10³/uL	1.5–6.6
Lymphocytes (pct)	42.0	Percent	18.0–48.3
Lymphocytes (ct)	2.5	×10³/uL	1.1–2.9

Test	Result	Units	Reference Ranges
Monocytes (pct)	10.4	Percent	4.4–12.7
Monocytes (ct)	0.8	×10³/uL	0.2–0.8
Eosinophils (pct)	4.7	Percent	0.6–7.3
Eosinophils (ct)	0.3	×10³/uL	0.0–0.4
Basophils (pct)	1.2	Percent	0.0–1.7
Basophils (ct)	0.1	×10³/uL	0.0–0.1

CMP—03/29/2017

Test	Result	Units	Reference Ranges
Sodium	134 (LO)	mmol/L	137–145
Potassium–serum	3.2 (LO)	mmol/L	3.6–5.2
Chloride	98 (LO)	mmol/L	100–110
Glucose	121 (HI)	mg/dL	60–100
BUN	22 (HI)	mg/dL	7–17
Creatinine	1.24 (HI)	mg/dL	0.52–1.04
Urea nitrogen/ Cr ratio	17.7	Ratio	
GFR	50	mL/minute	
Osmolality	278	mosm/kg	275–295
Uric acid	6.5 (HI)	mg/dL	2.5–6.2
Total protein	6.2 (LO)	g/dL	6.5–8.1
Albumin	2.7 (LO)	g/dL	3.2–4.4

(continues)

Test	Result	Units	Reference Ranges
Globulin	3.5	g/dL	2.7–4.3
Albumin/globulin ratio	0.77	Ratio	
Calcium	7.8 (LO)	mg/dL	8.4–10.2
Bilirubin	1.1	mg/dL	0.2–1.3
ALT	40	U/L	9–52
AST	22	U/L	14–36
Alkaline phosphatase	96	U/L	38–126

▶ Nursing Intake and Output Queries

03/28/2017

Intake				
	0000–0800 hrs	0800–1600 hrs	1600–2400 hrs	24-hour total
IV/FL		40 mL	40 mL	80 mL
PO	240 mL	360 mL	600 mL	1200 mL
Total	**240 mL**	**400 mL**	**640 mL**	**1,280 mL**

Output				
	0000–0800 hrs	0800–1600 hrs	1600–2400 hrs	24-hour total
Urine	400 mL	1,300 mL	1,500 mL	3,200 mL
BM		medium		
Total	**400 mL**	**1,300 mL**	**1,500 mL**	**3,200 mL**

24-hour total fluid balance: −1920 mL.

03/29/2017

Intake				
	0000–0800 hrs	0800–1600 hrs	1600–2400 hrs	24-hour total
IV/FL		40 mL		
PO	120 mL	240 mL		
Total	**120 mL**	**280 mL**		

Output				
	0000–0800 hrs	0800–1600 hrs	1600–2400 hrs	24-hour total
Urine	800 mL	780 mL		
BM	small			
Total	**800 mL**	**780 mL**		

Meal Record

	Breakfast	Snack	Lunch	Snack	Dinner	Snack	24-hour Total
03/28/2017	240 mL		360 mL		360 mL		960 mL—meals
03/29/2017	120 mL	10%	240 mL				

Weight Log

	03/28/2017	03/29/2017	03/30/2017	03/31/2017
Method	Bed Scale	Bed Scale		
Weight (lbs)	112	109		
Weight (kg)	50.9	49.5		
Height (in)	66			

▶ Resources

Evidenced-based practice guidelines, protocols, or algorithms used in creating scenarios include the following. Students may wish to review these resources in preparation for the simulation scenario.

- Kane and Prelack. *Advanced Medical Nutrition Therapy.* Jones & Bartlett Learning: Burlington, 2018.
- Academy of Nutrition and Dietetics. Evidence Based Practice Guidelines.
- Academy of Nutrition and Dietetics. Nutrition Care Manual.
- Safaii-Waite. *Medical Nutrition Therapy Simulations.* Online module: Chronic obstructive pulmonary disorder. Jones & Bartlett Learning: Burlington, 2017.

▶ Key Words

Bronchitis
Budesonide
Electroconvulsive therapy
Fluid retention
Inhalations
Lithium
Nares
Osmolality
Shallow breathing
Uric acid
Venofer
Wasting

SIMULATION SCENARIO:

Type 1 Diabetes Mellitus

LEARNING OBJECTIVES

- Identify different nutrition interventions for type 1 diabetes mellitus and how to select the appropriate intervention
- Identify the recommended nutrition therapy for patients with type 1 diabetes
- Estimate protein, calorie, and fluid needs for the patient
- Complete a dietary recall and assess adequacy of diet recall

▶ Student and Instructor Preparation

- Read chapter and lecture notes on medical nutrition therapy for type 1 diabetes mellitus
- Understand national MNT guidelines for this disease and potential risk factors, including: malnutrition, stress, unhealthy eating habits, smoking, alcohol consumption, age at diagnosis, and chronic diseases R/T diabetes
- Review Evidence Based Library of the Academy of Nutrition and Dietetics
- Review equations for estimation of energy, protein, and fluid needs for wound patients
- Practice online decision-tree module for type 1 diabetes mellitus

▶ Lab Set Up

Patient: Melissa Jones

Patient characteristics: Ms. Jones is a 21-year-old college student who lives in an apartment here in town while attending school. She has had type 1 diabetes mellitus for 5 years. She has had an insulin pump for 4 years and can manage her blood sugar well. She doesn't like vegetables and eats fast food often since it is quick; she also likes diet soda. She recently broke up with her boyfriend of 1 year and is emotionally stressed because of that, keeping up with school, and working a part-time job.

Environment/setting/location: Patient's Hospital Room/In-patient in ICU.

Lab staff needed on day of simulation: Preceptor/evaluator (1) or patient (1) (can be another preceptor/instructor, sim man, another student or actor), (1) can be another student.

Equipment, supplies, and prop list: Hospital room; curtain draped just inside door as privacy barrier; bed with pillow and blanket; chair at bedside; piece of paper to act as diet information handout, if desired; IV pole with bag of water hanging to act as IV fluids; cup of ice chips at bedside on bedside table.

▶ Clinical Case Information (02/23/2017)

Subjective

Ms. Jones is a 21-year-old female who is attending college and recently split with her boyfriend and has been under a tremendous amount of stress juggling her social life, school, work, and her type 1 diabetes mellitus. She presented to the ER this evening with nausea, vomiting, weakness, and abdominal pain. In addition to this, she has been getting up to use the bathroom quite often and reports burning during urination. She has an insulin pump and reports that she feels like she has been controlling her diabetes up until 2 days ago. She says she has been feeling ill but is not sure what is going on. She reports no fevers, cough, or headache. She is a little short of breath. Patient is reporting that she is tired and just wants to lay down and get some sleep.

Objective
Vital signs

- Blood pressure: 105/60
- Temperature: 101.8°F
- O_2: 91% on room air
- Respirations: 25–30/minute
- Pulse rate: 95 bpm
- Weight: 124 lbs
- Height: 5'1"

Meds

- Insulin Pump with Novolog (has Medtronic Paradigm 512) with basal rate of 0.8 units per hour and 7 units fast acting per meal. She states that she uses a correction factor of 1,800 for Humalog, if needed.
- Ca^{++} with vitamin D 500 mg/1,000 mg— 2 capsules daily
- Folic acid 400 µg daily
- MVI with minerals daily
- Valtrex 1,000 mg b.i.d. prn for cold sores
- Wellbutrin 300 mg daily

Abnormal lab values

- Serum Glucose 314 (high)
- pH 7.28 (low)
- Bicarb 17.5 mEq/L
- Beta-hydroxybutyrate (high)
- Positive for urine ketones
- Osmolality 310 (high)
- Anion Gap 13.0 (high)
- Na^+ 149
- K^+ 4.9
- BUN 20 (high)
- Cr 1.0

System review

- Heart: unremarkable, no dysrhythmia.
- Lungs: clear

- Extremities: Neurologically no concerns; no edema
- Chest: no rales or wheezing
- CV: decreased blood pressure
- Abdomen: Soft, tender with abdominal pain to lower quads.
- Neurologic: unremarkable; tiredness

Assessment/Plan

1. Appears to be early/mild DKA with classic signs and symptoms, including dehydration. Will order a UA to r/o sepsis from UTI. Certainly will look at r/o for other infectious illnesses. We will initiate IV fluids NaCl at 150 mL per hour, correct electrolytes, correct pH. Will discontinue her insulin pump for now and she will receive IV insulin within 1 hour after starting IV fluids along with D5 added to ensure a continuous insulin rate while glucose values slowly recover. Will initiate continuous IV insulin at 0.1 U/Kg/h. We will monitor Cl values and K^+ values closely as well as glucose. Follow for K^+ maintenance protocol.

2. UTI—suspected given patient c/o lower quadrant abdominal pain, urgency, and burning during urination. Follow-up with UA. Start ceftriaxone IV.

3. Acidosis—Related to #1, expect as a result of some underlying infection R/T #2.

4. Depression—Patient has been on Wellbutrin without problems, d/c this for now.

$1.267 \times 1.3 \times 1.3$

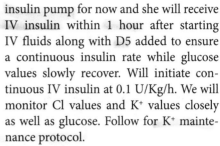

▸ Medication/Orders

Medication Orders	Amount	Route	Start Date
D5 IV	150 mL/hour	IV	02/23/2017
IV Insulin (regular) drip w/ 50 mL D5	5 U/hour	IV	02/23/2017
K^+ replacement	20 mEq/L	IV	02/23/2017
Ceftriaxone W/100 mL D5	1 gram	IV	02/23/2017
Calcium/vitamin D	500 mg/1,000 mg	p.o.	Hold
MVI with minerals	1 capsule daily	p.o.	Hold
Folic acid	400 µg	p.o.	Hold
Wellbutrin	300 mg daily	p.o.	Hold
Valtrex	1,000 mg b.i.d. prn	p.o.	Hold

Diet

NPO

Therapy Orders

R.D. consult for nutrition needs prn *unnecessary*
S.T. routine orders

▶ Physician Progress Note 02/24/2017

Subjective

Patient has responded well to insulin therapy in the past 24 hours. Her glucose is down to 200 mg/dL this a.m. and she is more alert. She is asking for something to drink this morning. If she continues to do well, we will consider advancing her diet later today.

Objective

Vital signs

- Blood pressure: stable at 120/80
- O_2: 93% on 1 L oxygen (will see if we can wean her off O_2)
- Weight: 124 lbs
- Height: 5'1"

Abnormal lab values

- Electrolytes normalized
- BUN 18 (high)
- Calcium 7.8 (low)

Meds

- IV Ceftriaxone (Rocephin)
- Regular insulin IV continuous rate
- IV fluids

Assessment/Plan

1. Early/mild DKA improving; we can probably switch to IM insulin and continue to monitor her glucose, anion gap, osmolality, and ketones.
2. UTI—UA shows 3+ bacteria, will continue with current Rocephin dose IV. Patient's nausea is improving; will try advancing diet and try to get her on oral ABX within the next 24 hours.
3. Acidosis—resolving.
4. Acute renal compromise—due to dehydration on admission, resolved.
5. Depression—We can restart her antidepressant as soon as she can tolerate her diet.
6. We will try to get patient up and ambulating today and advance her diet to clear liquids.

▶ Multidisciplinary Progress Notes

Nursing Progress Note 02/23/2017: 1700

Patient resting quietly in her room. No signs of distress noted. IV running at 150 mL per hour.

Nursing Progress Note 02/23/2017: 2245

Blood Pressure taken/vitals taken. Patient resting; has been sleeping since admission.

Social Services Progress Note 02/24/2017: 0945

Patient reports she is feeling a little better today; she says her family is on their way to see her from out of town, and her mother will stay with her for a few days until she feels better. Patient upset about breakup with boyfriend, but otherwise, pleasant today.

Nursing Progress Note 02/24/2017: 1115

Patient's ex-boyfriend attempted to visit her but she did not allow him to enter her room. Ex left, patient is in bed and upset regarding the incident. Notified Social Services. Blood pressure taken. 94% oxygen on room air.

Nursing Progress Note 02/24/2017: 1200

Patient's diet advanced to clear liquids; patient refused to order a tray. She is lying in bed, stating that she doesn't feel well and doesn't want to speak with anyone. Patient refused to get up to shower.

Nursing Progress Note 02/24/2017: 1300

Vitals taken, encouraged patient to try ordering a meal. She says she is not interested in eating today.

Nursing Progress Note 02/24/2017: 1615

Patient has been sleeping all afternoon. When entering the room, can see patient stirring, but she refuses to wake up when spoken to.

▶ Labs

CBC—02/23/2017

Test	Result	Units	Reference Ranges
WBC	12.0 (HI)	×10³/uL	4.8–10.8
RBC	5.50	×10³/uL	4.10–6.70
Hemoglobin	13.0	g/dL	12.5–16.0
Hematocrit	37.0	Percent	37.0–47.0
Erythrocyte MCV	90.8	fL	81.0–96.0
Erythrocyte MCH	36.6	pg	33.0–39.0
Erythrocyte MCHC	34.0	g/dL	32.0–36.0
RDW	18.5 (HI)	Percent	13.0–18.0
MPV	8.8	fL	6.9–10.6

(continues)

Test	Result	Units	Reference Ranges
Platelet count	360	×10³/uL	130–400
Neutrophils (pct)	88.0 (HI)	Percent	39.3–73.7
Neutrophils (ct)	7.0 (HI)	×10³/uL	1.5–6.6
Lymphocytes (pct)	67.2	Percent	18.0–48.3
Lymphocytes (ct)	2.3	×10³/uL	1.1–2.9
Monocytes (pct)	6.8	Percent	4.4–12.7
Monocytes (ct)	0.3	×10³/uL	0.2–0.8
Eosinophils (pct)	7.0	Percent	0.6–7.3
Eosinophils (ct)	0.4	×10³/uL	0.0–0.4
Basophils (pct)	0.5	Percent	0.0–1.7
Basophils (ct)	0.1	×10³/uL	0.0–0.1

CMP—02/23/2017

Test	Result	Units	Reference Ranges
Sodium	149 (HI)	mmol/L	137–145
Potassium–serum	5.0 (HI)	mmol/L	3.6–5.2
Chloride	111 (HI)	mmol/L	100–110
Glucose	314 (HI)	mg/dL	60–100
Osmolality	310 (HI)	mosm/kg	275–295
Anion gap	16.0	mEq/L	8–16 mEq/L
BUN	20 (HI)	mg/dL	7–17

Test	Result	Units	Reference Ranges
Creatinine	1.00	mg/dL	0.52–1.04
Urea nitrogen/Cr ratio	20	Ratio	
GFR	81	mL/minute	
Uric acid	5.0	mg/dL	2.5–6.2
Total protein	8.1	g/dL	6.5–8.1
Albumin	4.5 (HI)	g/dL	3.2–4.4
Globulin	3.59	g/dL	2.7–4.3
Albumin/globulin ratio	1.25	Ratio	
Calcium	9.0	mg/dL	8.4–10.2
Bilirubin	0.8	mg/dL	0.2–1.3
ALT	50	U/L	9–52
AST	30	U/L	14–36
Alkaline phosphatase	118	U/L	38–126
TSH	2.29	mIU/L	0.32–5.00

Capillary Glucose (Point of Care) 02/22/2017–02/23/2017: Time and Value

0800	1000	1200	1400	1600	1800
				299	290

2000	2200	2400	0200	0400	0600
276	266	240	233	223	212

Capillary Glucose (Point of Care) 02/23/2017–02/24/2017: Time and Value

0800	1000	1200	1400	1600	1800
205	200	198	190	187	
2000	2200	2400	0200	0400	0600

CBC—02/24/2017

Test	Result	Units	Reference Ranges
WBC	11.0 (HI)	×10³/uL	4.8–10.8
RBC	5.50	×10³/uL	4.10–6.70
Hemoglobin	12.6	g/dL	12.5–16.0
Hematocrit	37.0	Percent	37.0–47.0
Erythrocyte MCV	85.0	fL	81.0–96.0
Erythrocyte MCH	35.0	pg	33.0–39.0
Erythrocyte MCHC	33.5	g/dL	32.0–36.0
RDW	15.5	Percent	13.0–18.0
MPV	7.2	fL	6.9–10.6
Platelet count	225	×10³/uL	130–400
Neutrophils (pct)	45.2	Percent	39.3–73.7
Neutrophils (ct)	3.0	×10³/uL	1.5–6.6
Lymphocytes (pct)	40.1	Percent	18.0–48.3
Lymphocytes (ct)	2.0	×10³/uL	1.1–2.9

Test	Result	Units	Reference Ranges
Monocytes (pct)	6.7	Percent	4.4–12.7
Monocytes (ct)	0.4	×10³/uL	0.2–0.8
Eosinophils (pct)	3.3	Percent	0.6–7.3
Eosinophils (ct)	0.2	×10³/uL	0.0–0.4
Basophils (pct)	0.9	Percent	0.0–1.7
Basophils (ct)	0.0	×10³/uL	0.0–0.1

CMP—02/24/2017

Test	Result	Units	Reference Ranges
Sodium	140	mmol/L	137–145
Potassium–serum	3.6	mmol/L	3.6–5.2
Chloride	102	mmol/L	100–110
Glucose	200 (HI)	mg/dL	60–100
Osmolality	295	mosm/kg	275–295
BUN	18 (HI)	mg/dL	7–17
Creatinine	0.90	mg/dL	0.52–1.04
Urea nitrogen/ Cr ratio	20	Ratio	
Uric acid	6.0	mg/dL	2.5–6.2
Total protein	7.0	g/dL	6.5–8.1
Albumin	3.5	g/dL	3.2–4.4
Globulin	3.5	g/dL	2.7–4.3

(continues)

Test	Result	Units	Reference Ranges
Albumin/globulin ratio	1.00	Ratio	
Calcium	7.8 (LO)	mg/dL	8.4–10.2
Bilirubin	1.2	mg/dL	0.2–1.3
ALT	45	U/L	9–52
AST	25	U/L	14–36
Alkaline phosphatase	57	U/L	38–126

▶ Nursing Intake and Output Queries

02/23/2017

Intake				
	0000–0800 hrs	0800–1600 hrs	1600–2400 hrs	24-hour total
IV/FL			1,250 mL	1,250 mL
PO			NPO	NPO
Total			**1,250 mL**	**1,250 mL**

Output				
	0000–0800 hrs	0800–1600 hrs	1600–2400 hrs	24-hour total
Urine			600 mL	600 mL
BM				
Total			**600 mL**	**600 mL**

24-hour total fluid balance: 650 mL.

02/24/2017

Intake				
	0000–0800 hrs	0800–1600 hrs	1600–2400 hrs	24-hour total
IV/FL	1,200 mL	1,200 mL		
PO		50 mL		
Total	**1,200 mL**	**1,250 mL**		

Output				
	0000–0800 hrs	0800–1600 hrs	1600–2400 hrs	24-hour total
Urine	520 mL	530 mL		
BM				
Total	**520 mL**	**530 mL**		

Meal Record

	Breakfast	Snack	Lunch	Snack	Dinner	Snack	24-hour Total
02/23/2017	N/A		N/A		NPO	NPO	
02/22/2017	NPO		NPO	50 mL H_2O			

Weight Log

	02/23/2017	02/24/2017	02/25/2017	02/26/2017
Method	Bed Scale	Bed Scale		
Weight (lbs)	124	124		
Weight (kg)	56.3	56.3		
Height (in)	61			

▶ Resources

Evidenced-based practice guidelines, protocols, or algorithms used in creating scenarios include the following. Students may wish to review these resources in preparation for the simulation scenario.

- Kane and Prelack. *Advanced Medical Nutrition Therapy*. Jones & Bartlett Learning: Burlington, 2018.
- Academy of Nutrition and Dietetics. Evidence Based Practice Guidelines.
- Academy of Nutrition and Dietetics. Nutrition Care Manual.
- Academy of Nutrition and Dietetics. Academy of Nutrition and Dietetics Health Informatics Infrastructure (ANDHII). https://www.andhii.org/info/.
- Safaii-Waite. *Medical Nutrition Therapy Simulations*. Online module: Diabetes mellitus type 1. Jones & Bartlett Learning: Burlington, 2017.

▶ Key Words

Acidosis
DKA
Dysrhythmia
Humalog
IM Insulin
Novolog
Urine ketones
UTI
Wellbutrin

SIMULATION SCENARIO:

Type 2 Diabetes Mellitus

LEARNING OBJECTIVES

- Identify different nutrition interventions for type 2 diabetes mellitus and how to select the most appropriate intervention
- Be able to identify the recommended nutrition therapy for patients with type 2 diabetes
- Estimate protein, calorie, and fluid needs of the patient
- Complete a dietary recall/assessment the adequacy of diet recall

▶ Student and Instructor Preparation

- Read chapter and lecture notes on medical nutrition therapy for type 2 diabetes mellitus
- Understand national MNT guidelines for this disease, and potential risk factors, including stress, unhealthy eating habits, smoking, overweight or obesity, alcohol consumption, race, age, and chronic steroid use
- Review Evidence Based Library of the Academy of Nutrition and Dietetics
- Review equations for estimation of energy, protein, and fluid needs for wound patient
- Practice online decision-tree module for type 2 diabetes mellitus

▶ Lab Set Up

Patient: Carla Jenkins

Patient characteristics: Ms. Jenkins is a 50-year-old female with recently diagnosed type 2 diabetes mellitus. She was admitted to the hospital for a right total knee arthroplasty. She is a cook and does know a little about nutrition and carbohydrates. She wants to learn how to plan balanced meals to help control her blood sugar. She needs something basic because she doesn't have a lot of time to count carbohydrates.

Environment/setting/location: Hospital setting. The patient is s/p right knee arthroplasty.

Lab staff needed on day of simulation: Preceptor/evaluator (1) or patient (1) (can be another preceptor/instructor, sim man, another student, or actor).

Equipment, supplies, and prop list: Hospital room, bed, bedside table, and two chairs at bedside.

▶ Clinical Case Information (4/12/2017)

Subjective

Ms. Jenkins is a 50-year-old female who is here after consultation with her orthopedic surgeon, Dr. Weiss, for osteoarthritis of the right knee. She currently works as a cook for the elementary school near her house. She has complained of knee pain for several years and desired to have the knee replacement now as she will have PTO and has the summer off to recuperate before returning to work in the fall.

Objective

Vital signs

- Blood pressure: 140/79
- Temperature: 98.4°F
- O$_2$: 98% on room air
- Weight: 220 lbs
- Height: 5'2"

Meds

- Simvastatin 20 mg/day
- Metroprolol 12.5 mg twice daily

- Glimepiride 2 mg daily—started 1 month ago
- Levothyroxine 125 µg/day
- Fish Oil 1,000 mg capsule once daily
- MVI with minerals daily
- Vitamin D 2000 IU daily

Abnormal lab values

- Glucose 140 mg/dL—fasting
- BUN 25 (high)
- Cr 1.08 (high)
- Cholesterol 204 (high)
- Triglycerides 250 (high)
- Hgb A1c 7.5%
- Hgb A1c value from 1/30/13 found at 7.1%

Allergies

Penicillin (rash), bananas

Assessment

1. Osteoarthritis of the right knee per Dr. Weiss, orthopedic surgeon. Planned right total knee replacement next week.
2. Diabetes mellitus—started on glimepiride 2 mg daily p.o. on 3/10/2013.
3. Hypercholesterolemia—Carla is taking simvastatin 20 mg/day. We may need to increase this to 40 mg/day as her cholesterol and triglycerides are still above goal. Discontinue fish oil in preparation for surgery.
4. HTN—She remains on metroprolol 12.5 mg twice daily, which has been adequate.
5. Hypothyroidism—Will continue with current medication and dose.

Plan

Anticipate right total knee arthroplasty in 1 week by Dr. Weiss. Consult as needed s/p surgery. Follow-up with patient after surgery in 2 weeks for medical checkup and to discuss increase in her statin. May need to involve diabetic educator, as patient is a recently diagnosed diabetic, questionable as to what kind of education she has had concerning this.

▶ Physician Progress Note 04/12/2017

Subjective

Patient admitted to hospital s/p right TKA R/T hypotensive episode after surgery. Patient was given multiple boluses of IV fluids in attempts to improve blood pressure and they were successful in bringing her blood pressure up to an acceptable level. Patient is currently medically stable but will require observation for the next day or so, and for this reason, we will be admitting her to the surgical floor.

Objective

Vital signs

- Blood pressure: stable at 120/80
- O_2: 89% on 1 L oxygen
- Weight: 225 lbs

Abnormal lab values

- Na^+ 131 (low)
- Cl 98 (low)
- Glucose 132 (high)
- BUN 20 (high)
- Cr 1.05 (high)
- Total protein 6.4 (low)
- Calcium 8.0 (low)
- Hgb 12.0 (low)
- Hct 35.2 (low)

Meds

LR initially at 100 mL per hour, but now discontinued

- Simvastatin 20 mg/day
- Metroprolol 12.5 mg twice daily
- Glimepiride 2 mg daily
- Levothyroxine 125 µg/day
- MVI with minerals daily
- Vitamin D 2,000 IU daily

Allergies

Penicillin (rash), bananas

Assessment

1. Hypotensive episode s/p surgery—resolved. Will keep patient under observation for the next 24 to 48 hours; continue with regular home medications as likely resolved with fluid boluses.
2. Patient is s/p right total knee arthroplasty. She is working with P.T. and starting to get up and to ambulate. We will continue to have P.T. work with her.
3. Diabetes—Patient is on glimepiride. We will consult Nutrition to see if they can help with her diet and provide a calorie range for her to use at home.
4. Hypercholesterolemia—Increased her statin 1 week ago. We will continue this and check her lipid panel in 6 months.
5. Hypothyroid—No current issues. Continue with levothyroxine.
6. Renal insufficiency—Maybe R/T underlying diabetes just diagnosed. BUN and Cr slightly elevated; continue to monitor values.

▶ Medication/Orders

Medication Orders	Amount	Route	Start Date
Metroprolol	12.5 mg b.i.d.	p.o.	04/12/2017
Glimepiride	2 mg daily	p.o.	04/12/2017
Levothyroxine	125 µg daily	p.o.	04/12/2017
Simvastatin	20 mg/day	p.o.	04/12/2017
MVI with minerals	1 cap daily	p.o.	04/12/2017
Vitamin D 2000 IU daily	1 cap daily	p.o.	04/12/2017
Acetaminophen	325 mg q 6 hrs prn	p.o.	04/12/2017
Ondansetron	4–8 mg q 6 hrs prn	p.o.	04/12/2017
Simethicone	80 mg q 2 hrs prn	p.o.	04/12/2017
Lantus insulin	20 units q HS	IM	04/12/2017
Sliding scale Humalog	(Refer to low-dose SS Policy)		04/12/2017

Diet

NPO
Advance diet postsurgery, as tolerates
60 g/meal consistent carbohydrate

Therapy Orders

P.T. to ambulate twice daily, work with strengthening and balance.
R.D. consult for nutrition and diet needs prn.
S.T. consult prn.
Social Services consult with discharge planning for possible ECF placement for rehabilitation.

▶ Multidisciplinary Progress Notes

Social Services Consult/Discharge Planning Progress Note
04/12/2017: 0715

Patient and family in agreement that patient will go to Sea Side Care and Rehabilitation after discharge.

Nursing Progress Note
04/12/2017: 0730

Patient ordered breakfast this a.m., ate 100% but says she is still hungry. Patient given string cheese and crackers by R.N. 1 hour after breakfast.

Nursing Progress Note
04/12/2017: 1000

Patient resting quietly in bed, no s/s of distress. Vital signs taken.

Nursing Progress Note
04/12/2017: 1530

Patient ate lunch at 1230, 60 gm carbohydrate/meal. She requested a snack—Diet Pepsi and a bowl of fruit. Capillary glucose 179 mg/dL. Sliding scale administered per Low Dose Humalog Policy at lunch (1240).

Nursing Progress Note
04/12/2017: 1600

Patient declined to work with physical therapy this afternoon. Says she is tired.

▶ Labs

CBC—04/12/2017

Test	Result	Units	Reference Ranges
WBC	7.1	$\times 10^3$/uL	4.8–10.8
RBC	5.44	$\times 10^3$/uL	4.10–6.70
Hemoglobin	14.2	g/dL	12.5–16.0
Hematocrit	45.7	Percent	37.0–47.0
Erythrocyte MCV	85.5	fL	81.0–96.0
Erythrocyte MCH	29.2 (LO)	pg	33.0–39.0
Erythrocyte MCHC	31.9 (LO)	g/dL	32.0–36.0
RDW	13.5	Percent	13.0–18.0
MPV	7.2	fL	6.9–10.6
Platelet count	294	$\times 10^3$/uL	130–400

(continues)

Test	Result	Units	Reference Ranges
Neutrophils (pct)	49.4	Percent	39.3–73.7
Neutrophils (ct)	3.5	×10³/uL	1.5–6.6
Lymphocytes (pct)	43.5	Percent	18.0–48.3
Lymphocytes (ct)	2.8	×10³/uL	1.1–2.9
Monocytes (pct)	4.7	Percent	4.4–12.7
Monocytes (ct)	0.3	×10³/uL	0.2–0.8
Eosinophils (pct)	1.8	Percent	0.6–7.3
Eosinophils (ct)	0.1	×10³/uL	0.0–0.4
Basophils (pct)	0.7	Percent	0.0–1.7
Basophils (ct)	0.0	×10³/uL	0.0–0.1

CMP—04/12/2017

Test	Result	Units	Reference Ranges
Sodium	131 (LO)	mmol/L	137–145
Potassium–serum	3.6	mmol/L	3.6–5.2
Chloride–serum	98 (LO)	mmol/L	100–110
Glucose	132 (HI)	mg/dL	60–100
BUN	20 (HI)	mg/dL	7–17
Creatinine	1.05 (HI)	mg/dL	0.52–1.04
Urea nitrogen/Cr ratio	19.0	Ratio	
GFR	66	mL/minute	

Test	Result	Units	Reference Ranges
Uric acid	4.6	mg/dL	2.5–6.2
Total protein	6.4 (LO)	g/dL	6.5–8.1
Albumin	3.2	g/dL	3.2–4.4
Globulin	3.2	g/dL	2.7–4.3
Albumin/globulin ratio	1.0	Ratio	
Calcium	8.0 (LO)	mg/dL	8.4–10.2
Bilirubin	0.6	mg/dL	0.2–1.3
ALT	24	U/L	9–52
AST	16	U/L	14–36
Alkaline phosphatase	53	U/L	38–126
TSH	0.88	uIU/mL	0.32–5.00

BMP with Lipid Profile—04/12/2017

Test	Result	Units	Reference Ranges
Sodium	139	mmol/L	137–145
Potassium–serum	3.9	mmol/L	3.6–5.2
Chloride–serum	103	mmol/L	100–110
Glucose	140 (HI)	mg/dL	60–100
BUN	25 (HI)	mg/dL	7–17
Creatinine	1.08 (HI)	mg/dL	0.52–1.04
Chloride–serum	103	mmol/L	100–110

(continues)

Test	Result	Units	Reference Ranges
Glucose	140 (HI)	mg/dL	60–100
BUN	25 (HI)	mg/dL	7–17
Creatinine	1.08 (HI)	mg/dL	0.52–1.04
Calcium	9.3	mg/dL	8.4–10.2
Triglycerides	250	mg/dL	40–250
Cholesterol	204 (HI)	mg/dL	135–200
HDL cholesterol	34 (LO)	mg/dL	35–85
VLDL	32	mg/dL	7–38
LDL	137 (HI)	mg/dL	63–100
Total/HDL ratio	6.00 (HI)	Ratio	2.67–3.64
Hgb A1c	7.5 (HI)	Percent	<5.7

▶ Nursing Intake and Output Queries

04/12/2017

Intake				
	0000–0800 hrs	0800–1600 hrs	1600–2400 hrs	24-hour total
IV/FL	50 mL	50 mL	50 mL	150 mL
PO	800 mL	360 mL	660 mL	1,820 mL
PO		240 mL		240 mL
Total	**850 mL**	**650 mL**	**710 mL**	**2,210 mL**

Output				
	0000–0800 hrs	0800–1600 hrs	1600–2400 hrs	24-hour total
Urine	240 mL	180	240	660 mL
Urine	200 mL	360	300	860 mL
BM			50 mL	50 mL
Total	**440 mL**	**540 mL**	**590 mL**	**1,570 mL**

24-hour total fluid balance: 640 mL.

Meal Record

	Breakfast	Snack	Lunch	Snack	Dinner	Snack	24-hour Total
04/11/2017	NPO		NPO		500 mL		500 mL
04/12/2017	100%	100%	80%	100%	80%		86% average/ meal

Weight Log

	04/11/2017	04/12/2017	04/13/2017	04/14/2017
Method	**Bed Scale**	**Bed Scale**		
Weight (lbs)	221	225		
Weight (kg)	100.4	102.2		
Height (in)	62			

▶ Resources

Evidenced-based practice guidelines, protocols, or algorithms used in creating scenarios include the following. Students may wish to review these resources in preparation for the simulation scenario.

- Kane and Prelack. *Advanced Medical Nutrition Therapy*. Jones & Bartlett Learning: Burlington, 2018.
- Academy of Nutrition and Dietetics. Evidence Based Practice Guidelines.
- Academy of Nutrition and Dietetics. Nutrition Care Manual.
- Academy of Nutrition and Dietetics. Academy of Nutrition and Dietetics Health Informatics Infrastructure (ANDHII). https://www.andhii.org/info/.
- Safaii-Waite. *Medical Nutrition Therapy Simulations*. Online module: Diabetes mellitus type 2. Jones & Bartlett Learning: Burlington, 2017.

▶ Key Words

Arthroplasty
Glimepiride
Hypercholesterolemia
Hypotensive
NPO

SIMULATION SCENARIO:

Liver Disease

LEARNING OBJECTIVES

- Identify different nutrition interventions for liver disease and how to select the appropriate intervention
- Be able to identify the recommended nutrition therapy for patients with cirrhosis of the liver
- Estimate protein, calorie, and fluid needs for this patient

▶ Student and Instructor Preparation

- Read chapter and lecture notes on cirrhosis of the liver/liver disease
- Understand national MNT guidelines for cirrhosis and liver disease and potential risk factors, including malnutrition, stress, unhealthy eating habits, smoking, alcohol consumption, excessive fat intake, and chronic disease
- Review Evidence Based Library of the Academy of Nutrition and Dietetics
- Review equations for estimation of energy, protein, and fluid needs for a patient with liver disease
- Practice online decision-tree module for liver disease

▶ Lab Set Up

Patient: Frank Jimenez

Patient characteristics: Mr. Jimenez is a 65-year-old male who resides at a local, extended-care facility. He has an Hx of ETOH abuse, which has resulted in cirrhosis of the liver; he also suffers from the effects of a late CVA, which has left his right side paralyzed. He has difficulty feeding himself and he requires a mechanically altered diet. His alertness has been normal up until the day before he was admitted to the ER for decreased alertness and shortness of breath. He does not have good family support, as his four children are all married and live outside of the state; his wife passed away 2 years ago from a sudden heart attack. He is aphasic and communicates by nodding his head "yes" or "no."

Environment/setting/location: Patient's hospital room; nursing station outside of the patient's room.

Lab staff needed on day of simulation: Preceptor/evaluator (1) or patient (1) (can be another preceptor/instructor, sim man, another student or actor). Optional: student or actor as patient's nurse at end of scenario.

Equipment, supplies, and prop list: Hospital room, curtain draped just inside door as privacy barrier; bed with pillow and blanket; a flip chart or notebook to act as patient's chart; a chair and desk outside of the patient's room for nursing staff; infection control cart outside of the patient's room with disposable gloves, mask, and gown. Set up a garbage can inside patient's room to act as a receptacle for contaminated infection control clothing. Offer a bottle of hand sanitizer inside patient's room to help with learning proper infection control measures. Set up a desk with a chair and a notebook (to act as patient's chart) for "nurse's station."

▸ Clinical Case Information (05/05/2017)

Subjective

Mr. Jimenez is a man who has undoubtedly had a series of unfortunate events in the past 5 to 8 years of his life. He has an Hx of strong ETOH use, which has resulted in cirrhosis of the liver and, 5 years ago, he had a CVA, resulting in aphasia, dysphagia, and right-sided weakness. His wife of 45 years passed away 2 years ago from a sudden heart attack. He is a resident of a local ECF here in town, where he has lived for 5 years, essentially since he had the stroke. The staff there report that he has become more hypoxic and short of breath over the past couple of days. I am told that his intake has been poor for several weeks and that they think he has lost weight, although they are not sure how much. He is also becoming more confused and does not answer questions in his usual manner of shaking or nodding his head. The staff reports that he had an oxygen value of 80% this morning (he usually does not require O_2). The patient's primary doctor was contacted and he recommended that he be brought to the ER.

Objective
Vital signs

- Blood pressure: 141/82
- Temperature: 102.5°F
- O_2: 81% on room air, now requiring 2 Liters O_2, bringing O_2 up to 90%
- Respiration: 32 per minute
- Pulse rate: 88 beats per minute
- Weight: 180 lbs
- Height: 5'8"

PMHx

Allergic rhinitis, nonepileptic seizure disorder, A-fib, anxiety, HTN, cirrhosis of the liver r/t excessive ETOH use, debilitating headaches

Meds

- Cordarone 400 mg daily
- Propranolol 80 mg daily
- Lorazepam 2 mg daily
- Lopressor 100 mg daily
- Phenobarbitol 2 mg daily
- Rifaximin 550 mg daily
- Zocor 40 mg daily

- HCTZ 25 mg daily
- Lasix 40 mg daily
- Lactulose 15 mL daily
- Irbesartan 200 mg daily
- Cetirizine 10 mg daily prn
- Daily MVI with minerals
- Vitamin D 2000 IU daily
- Vitamin E 400 µg daily

Abnormal lab values

- Glucose 105 mg/dL (high)
- Osmolality 277 (low)
- BUN 24 (high)
- Calcium 7.9 (low)
- Sodium 133 (low)
- K$^+$ 3.3 (low)
- Magnesium 1.3 (low)
- Albumin 2.1 (low)
- AST 43 (high)
- ALT 66 (high)
- Bilirubin 2.4 (high)
- Hgb 10.0 (low)
- Hct 35.0 (low)
- Elevated neutrophils, lymphocytes, and slightly elevated eosinophils
- WBC 13.0 (high)
- Ammonia 50 (high)

System review

- Heart: Hx of dysrhythmia.
- Lungs: crackles bilateral lower lobe lungs.
- Extremities: 2+ edema to bilateral lower legs. Flaccid to right side due to CVA effects. Skin has a slight yellowish tinge. Physical exam reveals subcutaneous muscle wasting to scapular and clavicle regions consistent with severe malnutrition assessment guidelines.
- Chest: rapid, shallow, labored breathing. Vascular spider veins present.
- CV: lower extremity edema, elevated BP.
- Abdomen: hard mass to upper left quadrant, mild-to-moderate abdominal ascites, active bowel sounds.

- Neurologic: right side compromised, with dysphasia and aphasia Hx; currently with decreased alertness.

Assessment/Plan

1. Bilateral pneumonia—We will obtain a chest x-ray to help determine if this is viral vs bacterial. We will also consider aspiration pneumonia. He is requiring 2 liters of O$_2$ and maintaining oxygen levels at 90%. We will initiate IV antibiotics, including azithromycin and zosyn; follow up for result of x-ray.

2. Liver disease—Cirrhosis with link to ETOH use and portal hypertension. Due to decreased alertness, we will obtain an ammonia level again tomorrow. Question if patient has been refusing to take meds lately, including lactulose and Lasix. We will consider performing abdominal paracentesis to remove excess fluid buildup. Increase IV Lasix from 40 mg daily to 80 mg daily IV, hold on lactulose and we will avoid enemas until stool sample can be obtained. We will guaiac any stool to r/o GI bleeding from varices secondary to decreased Hgb and Hct values. Certainly, the reports of his decreased intake and potential weight loss are of concern. May consider an upper endoscopy if the patient is stable.

3. Malnutrition—Based on physical exam finding, including subcutaneous muscle wasting to scapula and clavicle regions, 2+ edema to bilateral lower extremities, ascites in abdominal region, unspecified amount of weight loss × 1 month or greater with intakes of 50% or less for at least 1 month.

4. A-fib—Currently on propranolol and cordarone. We will hold these for now until his respiratory compromise improves. We will initiate nicardipine at 5 mg/hr toward goal of 30 mg/hr. We will

continue to monitor BP and adjust the dose as needed.

5. Nonepileptic seizure disorder—On phenobarbital; will offer 40 mg every 12 hours IV for maintenance.

6. Anxiety—Hold oral med, offer 3.5 mg lorazepam every 12 hours prn.

7. HTN—BP elevated at 141/82, maintain on IV fluids of D5 at 75 mL per hour; continue to check every 4 hours. We will change lopressor p.o. to hydralazine IV 20 mg every 8 hours.

8. Dysphagia—The patient will be kept NPO for now.

▶ Medication/Orders

Medication Orders	Amount	Route	Start Date
D5	75 mL/hr	IV	05/05/2017
Azithromycin in NaCl 0.65%	500 mg/day 100 mL/hr	IV	05/05/2017
Zosyn in NaCl 0.65%	4.5 g/day 100 mL/hr	IV	05/05/2017
Ondansetron	4 mg every 6 hrs	IV	05/05/2017
Clopidogrel in NaCl	75 mg daily 100 mL	IV	05/05/2017
Simethicone	80 mg every 2 hrs	IV	05/05/2017
Promethazine	25 mg every 6 hrs	IV	05/05/2017
Furosemide	80 mg daily	IV	05/05/2017
Phenobarbitol	40 mg q 12 hrs	IV	05/05/2017
Lorazepam	3.5 mg q 12 hrs	IV	05/05/2017
Hydralazine	20 mg q 8 hrs	IV	05/05/2017
Nicardipine	5 mg per hour	IV	05/05/2017

Diet

NPO

Therapy Orders

R.D. consult for nutrition prn.
S.T. consult related to dysphagia when patient is more alert.
Social Services consult with discharge planning back to ECF for long-term care.

▶ Physician Progress Note 05/06/2017

Subjective

Mr. Jimenez presents this a.m. with somewhat improved mental status, but he is still having some confusion. He has received an IV antibiotic through the night and has had good urine output with IV Lasix. Speech therapy evaluation complete today and recommending a moist mechanical soft diet texture with nectar thick liquids. We will work on changing over to oral medications later today. Guaiac stool was negative yesterday, so we will probably hold off on endoscopy. Chest x-ray is consistent with viral pneumonia, however, it appears that he may have aspiration pneumonia to the left lower lobe as well. We will continue using IV antibiotics. Mr. Jimenez underwent abdominal paracentesis earlier and tolerated the procedure well with 4 liters of fluid removed. Patient's breathing is more relaxed but still requiring oxygen and IV antibiotics.

Objective

Vital signs

- Blood pressure: stable at 130/80
- O_2: 93% on 1 L oxygen; improved from 2 L yesterday

- Weight: 176 lbs, down 4 lbs from admission R/T to diuresis and 4 L paracentesis.

Abnormal lab values

- Na^+ 134 (low)
- K^+ 3.5 (low)
- Cl 98 (low)
- Glucose 100 (high)
- BUN 23 (high)
- Total protein 6.2 (low)
- Albumin 2.2 (low)
- Calcium 7.8 (low)
- ALT 64 (high)
- AST 43 (high)
- Hgb 10.8 (low)
- Hct 36.0 (low)
- WBC 11.6 (high)
- Ammonia 44 (WNL)

Meds

- D5 at 75 mL/hr
- Azithromycin 500 mg/day IV
- Zosyn 4.5 gm daily IV
- Ondansetron 4 mg q 6 hrs prn IV
- Clopidogrel 75 mg daily IV
- Simethicone 80 mg q 2 hrs prn IV
- Promethazine 25 mg q 6 hrs prn IV
- Furosemide 80 mg daily IV
- Phenobarbitol 40 mg q 12 hrs IV
- Lorazepam 3.5 mg q 12 hrs prn IV
- Hydralazine 20 mg q 8 hrs IV
- Nicardipine now at 25 mg/hr IV

Assessment/Plan

1. Viral pneumonia—bilateral with aspiration pneumonia to LLL. Continue with IV maintenance fluids, will try and obtain a speech evaluation today and increase oral diet. Continue with IV antibiotics. O_2 at 1 L; will also see if we can't reduce his O_2 needs today. Patient is on airborne precautions.

2. Cirrhosis of the liver—We will continue with IV Lasix today and see if we can't diurese him a little more. If diet is able to be advanced, will add lactulose regimen back into orders. Abdominal paracentesis successful 05/05/2017 with 4 liters fluid out. Negative stool guaiac 05/05/2017. Unsure regarding patient's diet at care facility, but definitely needs to be sodium restricted.
3. Malnutrition—We will seek a nutrition consult from the registered dietitian.
4. A-fib—We will see if we can't get him on his usual oral medications today.
5. Nonepileptic seizure disorder—Continue with same management.
6. Anxiety—Continues on lorazepam IV.
7. HTN—Continues on maintenance IV fluids, Lasix at 80 mg daily IV He will probably need a higher dose of Lasix when he goes back to the care facility and, with this, possibly some K^+ replacement. Would benefit from limiting sodium in his diet, as this certainly is a contributing factor to his fluid retention and him being uncomfortable.
8. Dysphagia—Follow speech therapy recommendations for diet textures.

▸ Multidisciplinary Progress Notes

Nursing Progress Note 05/05/2017: 1000

Patient resting quietly in bed. Breathing labored, maintaining oxygen on 2 L at 90%. I.V running at 75 mL per hour maintenance fluid. Catheter in place, 600 mL out this shift.

Nursing Progress Note 05/05/2017: 1200

BP taken 130/85. Patient had BM—soft medium, incontinent. Note orders to guaiac—negative result, physician notified. Continues resting in bed. Nasal cannula in place. Patient receiving IV fluids and IV antibiotics.

Nursing Progress Note 05/05/2017: 1430

Patient back from chest x-ray, IV restarted.

Social Services Consult 05/05/2017: 1600

Patient is from local ECF, expect planned return to care facility at discharge as bed held for patient.

Nursing Progress Note 05/06/2017: 0900

Patient waking for brief periods of time; is confused. He falls back asleep quickly. BP taken at 120/70, oxygen saturation 93% on 2 L O_2—Respiratory Therapy in and turned oxygen down to 1 L this a.m. Patient had 850 mL out last night.

Nursing Progress Note 05/06/2017: 1130

Bedside evaluation complete and S.T. recommends a moist, mechanical soft diet with nectar thick fluids. S.T. states swallow study would not be warranted at this point.

Nursing Progress Note 05/05/2017: 1230

Patient more alert at this hour but is still confused. Had small BM—continues to be incontinent. Physician wrote for abdominal paracentesis today at 1400. Edema 1+ LEs.

▶ Labs

CBC—05/05/2017

Test	Result	Units	Reference Ranges
WBC	13.0 (HI)	×10³/uL	4.8–10.8
RBC	4.80	×10³/uL	4.10–6.70
Hemoglobin	10.0 (LO)	g/dL	12.5–16.0
Hematocrit	35.0 (LO)	Percent	37.0–47.0
Erythrocyte MCV	81.0	fL	81.0–96.0
Erythrocyte MCH	34.0	pg	33.0–39.0
Erythrocyte MCHC	32.2	g/dL	32.0–36.0
RDW	14.0	Percent	13.0–18.0
MPV	7.1	fL	6.9–10.6
Platelet count	200	×10³/uL	130–400
Neutrophils (pct)	75.9 (HI)	Percent	39.3–73.7
Neutrophils (ct)	7.8 (HI)	×10³/uL	1.5–6.6
Lymphocytes (pct)	55.8 (HI)	Percent	18.0-48.3
Lymphocytes (ct)	3.9 (HI)	×10³/uL	1.1–2.9
Monocytes (pct)	4.7	Percent	4.4–12.7
Monocytes (ct)	0.4	×10³/uL	0.2–0.8
Eosinophils (pct)	7.4 (HI)	Percent	0.6–7.3
Eosinophils (ct)	0.4	×10³/uL	0.0–0.4
Basophils (pct)	1.0	Percent	0.0–1.7
Basophils (ct)	0.0	×10³/uL	0.0–0.1

CMP—05/05/2017

Test	Result	Units	Reference Ranges
Sodium	133 (LO)	mmol/L	137–145
Potassium–serum	3.3 (LO)	mmol/L	3.6–5.2
Chloride	100	mmol/L	100–110
Glucose	105 (HI)	mg/dL	60–100
BUN	24 (HI)	mg/dL	7–17
Creatinine	1.00	mg/dL	0.52–1.04
Magnesium	1.3 (LO)	mEq/L	1.5–2.5
Urea nitrogen/Cr ratio	26.7	Ratio	
GFR	79	mL/minute	
Osmolality	277 (LO)	mosm/kg	275–295
Uric acid	5.5	mg/dL	2.5–6.2
Total protein	6.0	g/dL	6.5–8.1
Albumin	2.1 (LO)	g/dL	3.2–4.4
Globulin	3.9	g/dL	2.7–4.3
Albumin/globulin ratio	0.53	Ratio	
Calcium	7.9 (LO)	mg/dL	8.4–10.2
Bilirubin	1.4 (HI)	mg/dL	0.2–1.3
ALT	66 (HI)	U/L	9–52
AST	43 (HI)	U/L	14–36
Alkaline phosphatase	126	U/L	38–126

Test	Result	Units	Reference Ranges
Ammonia	50 (HI)	µg/dL	15–45
Amylase	80	U/L	23–85
Lipase	155	U/L	0–160
TSH	4.20	mIU/L	0.32–5.00

CBC—05/06/2017

Test	Result	Units	Reference Ranges
WBC	11.6 (HI)	×10³/uL	4.8–10.8
RBC	5.06	×10³/uL	4.10–6.70
Hemoglobin	10.8 (LO)	g/dL	12.5–16.0
Hematocrit	36.0 (LO)	Percent	37.0–47.0
Erythrocyte MCV	80.1 (LO)	fL	81.0–96.0
Erythrocyte MCH	34.3	pg	33.0–39.0
Erythrocyte MCHC	31.1 (LO)	g/dL	32.0–36.0
RDW	13.9	Percent	13.0–18.0
MPV	7.5	fL	6.9–10.6
Platelet count	250	×10³/uL	130–400
Neutrophils (pct)	74.4 (HI)	Percent	39.3–73.7
Neutrophils (ct)	7.1 (HI)	×10³/uL	1.5–6.6
Lymphocytes (pct)	53.2 (HI)	Percent	18.0–48.3
Lymphocytes (ct)	3.2 (HI)	×10³/uL	1.1–2.9

(continues)

Test	Result	Units	Reference Ranges
Monocytes (pct)	7.2	Percent	4.4–12.7
Monocytes (ct)	0.6	×10³/uL	0.2–0.8
Eosinophils (pct)	7.3	Percent	0.6–7.3
Eosinophils (ct)	0.3	×10³/uL	0.0–0.4
Basophils (pct)	0.9	Percent	0.0–1.7
Basophils (ct)	0.0	×10³/uL	0.0–0.1

CMP—05/06/2017

Test	Result	Units	Reference Ranges
Sodium	134 (LO)	mmol/L	137–145
Potassium–serum	3.5 (LO)	mmol/L	3.6–5.2
Chloride	98 (LO)	mmol/L	100–110
Glucose	100 (HI)	mg/dL	60–100
BUN	23 (HI)	mg/dL	7–17
Creatinine	1.01 (HI)	mg/dL	0.52–1.04
Urea nitrogen/ Cr ratio	22.8	Ratio	
GFR	78	mL/minute	
Uric acid	5.7	mg/dL	2.5–6.2
Total protein	6.2 (LO)	g/dL	6.5–8.1
Albumin	2.2 (LO)	g/dL	3.2–4.4
Globulin	4.0	g/dL	2.7–4.3
Albumin/globulin ratio	0.55	Ratio	

Test	Result	Units	Reference Ranges
Calcium	7.8 (LO)	mg/dL	8.4–10.2
Bilirubin	1.3	mg/dL	0.2–1.3
ALT	64 (HI)	U/L	9–52
AST	43 (HI)	U/L	14–36
Alkaline phosphatase	120	U/L	38–126
Ammonia	44	µg/dL	15–45

▶ Nursing Intake and Output Queries

05/05/2017

Intake				
	0000–0800 hrs	0800–1600 hrs	1600–2400 hrs	24-hour total
IV/FL		900 mL	800 mL	1,700 mL
PO		NPO	NPO	NPO
Total		**900 mL**	**800 mL**	**1,700 mL**

Output				
	0000–0800 hrs	0800–1600 hrs	1600–2400 hrs	24-hour total
Urine	600 mL	800 mL	850 mL	2,250 mL
BM		Medium–solid/ soft		
Total	**600 mL**	**800 mL**	**850 mL**	**2,250 mL**

24-hour total fluid balance: −550 mL.

05/06/2017

Intake				
	0000–0800 hrs	0800–1600 hrs	1600–2400 hrs	24-hour total
IV/FL	600 mL	900 mL	800 mL	2,300 mL
PO	NPO	NPO	120 mL	120 mL
Total	**600 mL**	**900 mL**	**920 mL**	**2,420 mL**

Output				
	0000–0800 hrs	0800–1600 hrs	1600–2400 hrs	24-hour total
Urine	850 mL	1,000 mL	5,100 mL	6,950 mL
BM		Medium–solid/ soft		
Total	**850 mL**	**1,000 mL**	**5,100 mL**	**6,950 mL**

24 hour total fluid balance: −4,530 mL.

Meal Record

	Breakfast	Snack	Lunch	Snack	Dinner	Snack	24-hour Total
05/05/2017	N/A		NPO		NPO		NPO
05/06/2017	NPO		NPO		120 mL		120 mL
05/07/2017	30%						

Weight Log

	05/05/2017	05/06/2017	05/07/2017	05/08/2017
Method	Bed Scale	Bed Scale	Bed Scale	
Weight (lbs)	180	176	174	
Weight (kg)	81.8	80.0	79.0	
Height (in)	68			

▶ Resources

Evidenced-based practice guidelines, protocols, or algorithms used in creating scenarios include the following. Students may wish to review these resources in preparation for the simulation scenario.

- Kane and Prelack. *Advanced Medical Nutrition Therapy.* Jones & Bartlett Learning: Burlington, 2018.
- Academy of Nutrition and Dietetics. Evidence Based Practice Guidelines.
- Academy of Nutrition and Dietetics. Nutrition Care Manual.
- Safaii-Waite. *Medical Nutrition Therapy Simulations.* Online module: Liver disease. Jones & Bartlett Learning: Burlington, 2017.

▶ Key Words

Abdominal paracentesis
Ammonia
Aphasia
Cirrhosis
CVA
Dysphagia
ETOH
Flaccid
Guaiac
Paralyzed
Phenobarbital
Spider veins

SIMULATION SCENARIO:

Lung Cancer

LEARNING OBJECTIVES

- Identify different nutrition interventions for cancer patients and how to select the most appropriate intervention
- Be able to identify the recommended nutrition therapy for patients with cancer
- Estimate protein, calorie, and fluid needs for this patient

▶ Student and Instructor Preparation

- Read chapter and lecture notes on cancer
- Understand national MNT guidelines for this disease and potential risk factors, including: stress, unhealthy eating habits, smoking, overweight or obesity, alcohol consumption, race, heredity, and environmental factors
- Review Evidence Based Library of the Academy of Nutrition and Dietetics
- Review equations for estimation of energy, protein, and fluid needs for adults
- Practice decision-tree module for lung cancer

▶ Lab Set Up

Patient: Paul Couch

Patient characteristics: Paul is a 60-year-old male with end-stage lung cancer who has been receiving chemotherapy for the third time. He has been on disability for a year; he worked most of his life as a mechanic. He is married and has one son who lives 30 minutes away. Paul is tired and weak. He is unsure about how aggressively he wants to fight this disease. His family is hopeful that he will recover; however, Paul is physically exhausted and in pain.

Environment/setting/location: Hospital setting. This patient was admitted for pain management on the hospital medical floor.

Lab staff needed on day of simulation: Preceptor/evaluator (1) or patient (1) (can be another preceptor/instructor, sim man, another student or actor).

Equipment, supplies, and prop list: Hospital room, curtain hung to ensure patient privacy, hospital bed and bedding, bedside table, water jug on table at bedside.

▶ Clinical Case Information (04/10/2017)

Subjective

Paul is a 60-year-old male with lung cancer who just finished his third round of chemotherapy. He presented to the ER early this morning with severe pain issues, which have not been manageable at home r/t his cancer. He has been unable to eat for several days and reports that his appetite has been quite poor through this last round of chemotherapy and he has been drinking three to four Ensure nutrition supplements daily to try and meet his nutritional needs. He says he eats very little of anything else. He is noted to have severe malnutrition. He has been on supplemental enteral nutrition twice in the past year and a half due to his inability to consume adequate energy. His current outlook appears grim. He has been admitted for pain management several times in 3 months. With each admission, Paul continues to decline. We may need to consider end-of-life interventions and consult with Social Services and help him through this process, if the patient and family are in agreement.

Objective
Vital signs

- Blood pressure: 115/70
- Temperature: 101.5°F
- O_2: 90% on room air, now 93% on 1 L O_2
- Weight: 142 lbs
- Height: 5'9"
- UBW: 195 lbs
- BMI: 21.0 (WNL)
- Weight (6 months ago): 186 lbs (23.6%: severe).
- Physical assessment reveals severe subcutaneous fat loss to temporal, clavicle, scapular, and rib regions. Intake < 50% of normal for the past 3 to 6 months. Edema—2+ to lower extremities.

Meds

- Duragesic patch 25 µg/hr q 72 hours
- Acetaminophen 1,000 mg q 6 hours prn
- Aspirin 81 mg daily
- Prednisone 20 mg daily
- Amitriptyline 25 mg daily
- Zyloprim 100 mg daily
- Simvastatin 40 mg daily
- B-12 injection 1,000 µg monthly
- Mirtazapine 15 mg daily
- Tamsulosin 0.4 mg daily

Abnormal lab values

- WBC 6.2
- Hgb 9.6 (low)
- Hct 30.0 (low)
- MCV 77.0 (low)
- MCH 30.0 (low)
- MCHC 28.0 (low)
- RDW 12.6 (low)
- Neutrophils 37.5 (low)
- Total protein 6.3 (low)
- Albumin 2.7 (low)
- Osmolality 270 (low)
- Na^+ 134 (low)

- K⁺ 3.1 (low)
- Cl 97 (low)
- Calcium 7.4 (low)
- Serum iron 20 (low)
- Ferritin 8 (low)
- % Saturation 166 (low)
- TIBC 102 (high)

PMHx

Heart attack 2007 with CABG, GERD with esophageal erosion, B-12 deficiency, neutropenia, neutropenic colitis, *Helicobacter pylori*, benign prostatic hypertrophy, gout.

Family Hx

Father with prostate Ca, heart disease, COPD, GERD. Mother with HTN, hyperlipidemia.

Allergies

Sulfa, peanuts

Assessment

1. End-stage lung cancer—Paul has been admitted for pain management. We will discontinue oral pain medications and start methadone at 100 mL per hour. Due to continued decline and malnutrition, we will seek clarification regarding end-of-life decisions with Social Services as soon as the patient's family is available. We will also discuss the patient's desires regarding nutrition support as he has been on tube feedings in the past. He has been on mirtazapine, but without noticeable increase in intake.

2. Elevated temperature and dyspnea—It is quite possible that the patient has an underlying respiratory infection. We will start him on both Zosyn and azithromycin IV and will obtain a chest x-ray.

3. Anemia vs iron deficiency—We will give two units PRBC today.

4. Malnutrition—Related to #1, the patient has had poor intake for many months. We

will consult Clinical Nutrition to assist with evaluation of nutritional needs and follow to determine the patient's desire for nutrition support, if indeed it comes to that point.

5. Heart disease and past heart surgery—Patient continues on simvastatin and aspirin. We will start IV Lasix 40 mg b.i.d.

6. Benign prostatic hypertrophy—Continues on tamulosin.

7. Vitamin B-12 deficiency—Continues on vitamin B-12 injections IM monthly.

▶ Physician Progress Note 04/11/2017

Subjective

Paul says he slept better last night and states his pain, although severe, is better managed. He is tired and prefers to sleep or watch T.V. He is not interested in eating. He is still struggling with poor intake. As far as end-of-life interventions go, the patient is unsure that he wants to make a decision as this time. He says his wife is quite hopeful that he will recover despite multiple conversations with her regarding the patient's grim outlook. Chest x-ray revealed what appears to be an acute viral infection, suggesting bronchial pneumonia in addition to lung cancer. We will continue to cover with IV antibiotics for any underlying bacterial infection and manage symptoms. Certainly, nutrition is a concern. If Paul does not start eating in the next 24 hours, we will probably need to consider nutrition support as we have done in the past since he is not willing to choose advance directives for end-of-life care at this time.

Objective

Vital signs

- Blood pressure: stable at 112/68
- O₂: 91% on 1 L oxygen
- Weight: 141 lbs
- Temperature: 99.5°F

Abnormal lab values

- Hgb 10.8 (low)
- MCH 31.4 (low)
- MCHC 30.8 (low)
- Neutrophils 38.9 (low)
- Na^+ 136 (low)
- Osmolality 280
- Calcium 7.8 (low)
- Total protein 6.3 (low)
- Albumin 2.8 (low)

Meds

- Acetaminophen 1,000 mg q 6 hours prn
- Aspirin 81 mg daily
- Prednisone 20 mg daily
- Amitriptyline 25 mg daily
- Zyloprim 100 mg daily
- Simvastatin 40 mg daily
- Vitamin B-12 injection 1,000 µg monthly
- Mirtazapine 15 mg daily
- Tamsulosin 0.4 mg daily
- IV Zosyn and IV azithromycin
- Lasix 40 mg b.i.d

Allergies

Sulfa, peanuts

Assessment

1. End-stage lung cancer—Paul has been admitted for pain management. He is responding well to methadone at 100 mL per hour. He is still requiring acetaminophen q 6 hours for breakthrough pain and he rates his pain at a 4 out of 10.
2. Elevated temperature and dyspnea—Chest x-ray indicative of viral bronchitis, which is exacerbating lung cancer and resulting in increased pain issues and some hypoxia. Paul is doing well on 1 L O_2 with an average of 91% saturation.
3. Malnutrition—Paul is not eating well. He has been on a regular diet or whatever he will eat. Social Services consulted to discuss end-of-life decisions with the patient and his wife, who both state that they are not ready to make a decision. The patient is open to enteral nutrition if his appetite continues to be poor in the next 24 to 48 hours; however, he states that he does not want an NG tube as he has had this in the past. We will continue sending Ensure t.i.d. as the patient desires. He is drinking this, but little food intake.
4. Heart disease and past heart surgery—The patient continues on simvastatin and aspirin. We will continue with IV Lasix 40 mg b.i.d. and transition to Lasix p.o.
5. Benign prostatic hypertrophy—Continues on tamulosin.
6. Vitamin B-12 deficiency—Continues on B-12 injections IM monthly. He certainly needs to be evaluated for additional deficiencies, including iron deficiency and folic acid.

▶ Medication/Orders

Medication Orders	Amount	Route	Start Date
Acetaminophen	1,000 mg q 6 hrs	p.o.	04/10/2017
Aspirin	81 mg daily	p.o.	04/10/2017

(continues)

Medication Orders	Amount	Route	Start Date
Prednisone	20 mg daily	p.o.	04/10/2017
Simvastatin	20 mg/day	p.o.	04/10/2017
Amitriptyline	25 mg daily	p.o.	04/10/2017
Tamsulosin	0.4 mg daily	p.o.	04/10/2017
Mirtazapine	15 mg daily	p.o.	04/10/2017
Vitamin B-12	1,000 μg q month	IM	04/10/2017
Zosyn		IV	04/10/2017
Azithromycin		IV	04/10/2017
Furosemide	40 mg b.i.d.	IV	04/10/2017
PRBC	2 units	IV transfusion	04/10/2017

Diet

Regular
Ensure 8 oz. nutrition supplement t.i.d.

Therapy Orders

P.T. to ambulate twice daily, work on strengthening and balance.
R.D. consult for nutrition and diet needs; evaluate for nutrition support needs and route.
S.T. consult prn.
Social Services consult for possible end-of-life care.

▶ Multidisciplinary Progress Notes

Social Services Consult/Discharge Planning Progress Note 04/10/2017: 1100

Social Services visited with patient and family to discuss possible hospice. The patient and family wish to continue with same plan of care at this time and decline hospice measures. The patient reports he prefers to be a full code and still wants IV therapy/fluid and nutrition support, if necessary. Reviewed POLST form with patient and family. It was signed, dated, and is located in the chart.

Addendum—04/10/2017 1145: The patient's family left and the patient requested to speak with Social Services again. The patient reports that although he, personally, would consider hospice at this point, his spouse is having a very difficult time making that decision and he feels that she would feel responsible for his death if they chose hospice. The patient reports that his wife feels like they need to continue trying to beat this disease and she "doesn't want to give up on me."

Nursing Progress Note
04/10/2017: 1130

The patient was encouraged to order lunch, but he refused. He requested to drink a chocolate Ensure Plus. BP WNL 120/80. Oxygen at 93% on 1 L, Respiratory Therapy in to turn O_2 down to half a liter. IV ABX running according to orders without signs or symptoms of poor tolerance. Continuing to monitor.

Nursing Progress Note
04/10/2017: 1400

The patient resting quietly in bed. Continues to receive IV pain management. Patient reports pain at 4 out of 10. Family still out of facility. Patient encouraged to drink water at bedside. Patient reports some concerns with diarrhea over the past several months.

Nursing Progress Note
04/10/2017: 2100

Patient continues to have poor appetite. He drank two strawberry Ensures this eve. He did order dinner at nurse's request—a banana milkshake. Patient accepted about 50%, then vomited about 120 mL, saying he "felt full." IV pain management per orders, IV ABX per orders. O_2 decreased to room air with oxygen saturation at 92%. Patient states he is comfortable at this time.

Nursing Progress Note
04/11/2017: 0845

Patient up to work with physical therapist this a.m. and ambulated well. Patient now back in his bedroom and is tired. Encouraged patient to order breakfast. Patient ordered a bowl of melon and ate three bites. He accepted 120 mL of Ensure as well. Patient reports pain at 3 out of 10. Family here and at bedside. Patient reports bout of diarrhea this a.m. after eating breakfast.

Nursing Progress Note
04/11/2017: 0930

M.D. in to speak with the patient regarding his intake, which is poor and resulting in weight loss. Patient states that he is trying his best but that he gets full quickly. Continuing to offer Ensure, as the patient requests. Vital signs taken and oral meds given without problems.

▶ Labs

CBC—04/10/2017

Test	Result	Units	Reference Ranges
WBC	6.2	×10³/uL	4.8–10.8
RBC	4.4	×10³/uL	4.10–6.70
Hemoglobin	9.6 (LO)	g/dL	12.5–16.0
Hematocrit	30.0 (LO)	Percent	37.0–47.0
Erythrocyte MCV	77.0 (LO)	fL	81.0–96.0
Erythrocyte MCH	30.0 (LO)	pg	33.0–39.0
Erythrocyte MCHC	28.0 (LO)	g/dL	32.0–36.0
RDW	12.6 (LO)	Percent	13.0–18.0
MPV	6.9	fL	6.9–10.6
Platelet count	170	×10³/uL	130–400
Neutrophils (pct)	37.5 (LO)	Percent	39.3–73.7
Neutrophils (ct)	1.2 (LO)	×10³/uL	1.5–6.6
Lymphocytes (pct)	18.2	Percent	18.0–48.3
Lymphocytes (ct)	1.3	×10³/uL	1.1–2.9
Monocytes (pct)	4.8	Percent	4.4–12.7
Monocytes (ct)	0.4	×10³/uL	0.2–0.8
Eosinophils (pct)	2.8	Percent	0.6–7.3
Eosinophils (ct)	0.1	×10³/uL	0.0–0.4
Basophils (pct)	0.0	Percent	0.0–1.7
Basophils (ct)	0.0	×10³/uL	0.0–0.1

		Units	Reference Ranges
		mmol/L	137–145
		mmol/L	3.6–5.2
		mmol/L	100–110
		mg/dL	60–100
		mg/dL	7–17
		mg/dL	0.52–1.04
		Ratio	
		mL/minute	
Osmolality	270 (LO)	mosm/kg	275–295
Uric acid	2.7	mg/dL	2.5–6.2
Total protein	6.3 (LO)	g/dL	6.5–8.1
Albumin	2.7 (LO)	g/dL	3.2–4.4
Globulin	3.59	g/dL	2.7–4.3
Albumin/globulin ratio	0.75	Ratio	
Calcium	7.4 (LO)	mg/dL	8.4–10.2
Bilirubin	0.3	mg/dL	0.2–1.3
ALT	22	U/L	9–52
AST	27	U/L	14–36
Alkaline phosphatase	55	U/L	38–126
Amylase	60	U/L	23–85
Lipase	100	U/L	0–160

(continues)

Test	Result	Units	Reference Ranges
Serum iron	20 (LO)	µg/dL	30–170
Ferritin	8 (LO)	ng/mL	12–150
% saturation	166 (LO)	mg/dL	200–350
TIBC	102 (HI)	µmol/L	45–85
Serum folate	36.2	nmol/L	4.5–45.3

CBC—04/11/2017

Test	Result	Units	Reference Ranges
WBC	8.9	×10³/uL	4.8–10.8
RBC	5.6	×10³/uL	4.10–6.70
Hemoglobin	10.8 (LO)	g/dL	12.5–16.0
Hematocrit	37.2	Percent	37.0–47.0
Erythrocyte MCV	82.0	fL	81.0–96.0
Erythrocyte MCH	31.4 (LO)	pg	33.0–39.0
Erythrocyte MCHC	30.8 (LO)	g/dL	32.0–36.0
RDW	13.7	Percent	13.0–18.0
MPV	7.3	fL	6.9–10.6
Platelet count	275	×10³/uL	130–400
Neutrophils (pct)	38.9 (LO)	Percent	39.3–73.7
Neutrophils (ct)	1.4 (LO)	×10³/uL	1.5–6.6
Lymphocytes (pct)	25.6	Percent	18.0–48.3

Test	Result	Units	Reference Ranges
Lymphocytes (ct)	2.0	×10³/uL	1.1–2.9
Monocytes (pct)	5.7	Percent	4.4–12.7
Monocytes (ct)	0.5	×10³/uL	0.2–0.8
Eosinophils (pct)	6.3	Percent	0.6–7.3
Eosinophils (ct)	0.3	×10³/uL	0.0–0.4
Basophils (pct)	0.5	Percent	0.0–1.7
Basophils (ct)	0.0	×10³/uL	0.0–0.1

CMP—04/11/2017

Test	Result	Units	Reference Ranges
Sodium	136 (LO)	mmol/L	137–145
Potassium–serum	3.6	mmol/L	3.6–5.2
Chloride	101	mmol/L	100–110
Glucose	78	mg/dL	60–100
BUN	9	mg/dL	7–17
Creatinine	0.68	mg/dL	0.52–1.04
Urea nitrogen/ Cr ratio	13.2	Ratio	
GFR	>90	mL/minute	
Osmolality	280	mosm/kg	275–295
Uric acid	3.0	mg/dL	2.5–6.2
Total protein	6.3 (LO)	g/dL	6.5–8.1

(continues)

Test	Result	Units	Reference Ranges
Albumin	2.8 (LO)	g/dL	3.2–4.4
Globulin	3.8	g/dL	2.7–4.3
Albumin/globulin ratio	0.65	Ratio	
Calcium	7.8 (LO)	mg/dL	8.4–10.2

▶ Nursing Intake and Output Queries

04/10/2017

Intake				
	0000–0800 hrs	0800–1600 hrs	1600–2400 hrs	24-hour total
IV/FL	300 mL	1,075 mL	1,075 mL	2,450 mL
PO	120 mL	200 mL	480 mL	800 mL
Total	**420 mL**	**1,275 mL**	**1,555 mL**	**3,250 mL**

Output				
	0000–0800 hrs	0800–1600 hrs	1600–2400 hrs	24-hour total
Urine	360 mL	1,250 mL	900 mL	2,510 mL
BM			400 mL	400 mL
Emesis			120 mL	120 mL
Total	**360 mL**	**1,250 mL**	**1,420 mL**	**3,030 mL**

24-hour total fluid balance: 220 mL.

04/11/2017

Intake				
	0000–0800 hrs	0800–1600 hrs	1600–2400 hrs	24-hour total
IV/FL	150 mL	150 mL		
PO	120 mL	180 mL		
Total	**270 mL**	**330 mL**		

Output				
	0000–0800 hrs	0800–1600 hrs	1600–2400 hrs	24-hour total
Urine	600 mL	940 mL		
BM		200 mL		
Emesis				
Total	**600 mL**	**1,140 mL**		

Meal Record

	Breakfast	Snack	Lunch	Snack	Dinner	Snack	24-hour Total
04/11/2017	Declined	120 mL	Declined	200 mL	240 mL 50%	Declined	560 mL
04/12/2017	5%, 120 mL	N/A	10%, 240 mL				
04/13/2017							

Weight Log

	04/10/2017	04/11/2017	04/12/2017	04/13/2017
Method	Bed Scale	Bed Scale		
Weight (lbs)	142	141		
Weight (kg)	64.5	64.0		
Height (in)	69			

▶ Resources

Evidenced-based practice guidelines, protocols, or algorithms used in creating scenarios include the following. Students may wish to review these resources in preparation for the simulation scenario.

- Kane and Prelack. *Advanced Medical Nutrition Therapy.* Jones & Bartlett Learning: Burlington, 2018.
- Academy of Nutrition and Dietetics. Evidence Based Practice Guidelines.
- Academy of Nutrition and Dietetics. Nutrition Care Manual.
- Safaii-Waite. *Medical Nutrition Therapy Simulations.* Online module: Lung cancer. Jones & Bartlett Learning: Burlington, 2017.

▶ Key Words

Cancer
Chemotherapy
Colitis
Duragesic
Dyspnea
Hospice
Mirtazapine
Neutropenia
Nutrition Support
POLST

Acute Pancreatitis

LEARNING OBJECTIVES

- Identify different nutrition interventions for acute pancreatitis and how to select the appropriate intervention
- Be able to identify the recommended nutrition therapy for patients with acute pancreatitis
- Estimate protein, calorie, and fluid needs for patient in this scenario

▶ Student and Instructor Preparation

- Read chapter and lecture notes on medical nutrition therapy for acute pancreatitis
- Understand national MNT guidelines for this disease and potential risk factors, including: malnutrition, stress, unhealthy eating habits, smoking, alcohol consumption, gallbladder disease, and trauma
- Review Evidence Based Library of the Academy of Nutrition and Dietetics
- Review equations for estimation of energy, protein, and fluid needs for the patient
- Practice online decision-tree module for acute pancreatitis

▶ Lab Set Up

Patient/Sim Man/Actor Name: Suzie Jenkins

Patient characteristics: Mrs. Jenkins is a 45-year-old female with an Hx of gallstones. She is married with two children, who are both in college. She works full time at the local grocery store in the deli department. She tries to eat healthy, but goes out to eat with her husband on the weekends. They will usually get a steak or a gourmet hamburger with an alcoholic beverage. She has lost 10 lbs in the past couple of months related to decreased appetite and pain after eating in the upper abdomen, which radiates to her back. Although Suzie is overweight at 5'5" and 165 lbs, she does try to be active and participates in a bowling league several times a week.

She finds it difficult to stay on a meal plan while participating in her bowling league, since she often drinks a beer and snacks on fries while bowling with her friends.

Environment/setting/location: Patient's hospital room/in-patient on the med-surg floor.

Lab staff needed on day of simulation: Preceptor/evaluator (1) or patient (1) (can be another preceptor/instructor, sim man, another student or actor), (1) can be another student. (1) another student or actor for registered nurse.

Equipment, supplies, and prop list: Hospital room; curtain draped just inside door as privacy barrier; bed with pillow and blanket; chair at bedside; piece of paper to act as diet information handout, if desired; IV pole with a bag of water hanging to act as IV fluids; desk outside of patient's room with chair, pen, and flip chart.

▶ Clinical Case Information (02/23/2017)

Subjective

Mrs. Jenkins is a 45-year-old female with a Hx of gallstones several years ago. She comes into the ER with complaints of abdominal pain radiating to her back after she eats for the past several weeks. She says that she and her husband went out to eat and she started having these pains again. Pain appears to be in the epigastric and right upper quadrant areas. She is nauseated and has been vomiting. She denies smoking but drinks alcohol several times a week. She says her stools have been pasty looking. Her husband is here with her and she says she has good family support.

Objective
Vital signs

- Blood pressure: 111/70
- Temperature: 98.4°F
- O_2: 95% on room air
- Weight: 165 lbs
- Height: 5'5"
- UBW: 175 lbs

PMHx

Depression, hyperlipidemia, fibromyalgia, irritable bowel syndrome, gastroesophageal reflux disease (GERD), hypothyroidism, gallstones (did not require surgical intervention).

Past surgical Hx

Bilateral carpal tunnel surgery 2004, C-section × two: 1989 and 1992.

Family Hx

Father with type 2 diabetes mellitus, HTN, and gout. Mother with elevated cholesterol
Maternal grandmother with type 2 diabetes mellitus and HTN. Paternal grandfather deceased from CVA complications.

Meds

- Levothyroxine 75 µg daily
- Ca^{++} with vitamin D: two capsules daily
- Prevacid 30 mg daily
- Zoloft 25 mg daily
- Daily MVI with minerals
- Simvastatin 20 mg daily
- Bentyl 20 mg daily

Abnormal lab values

- BUN 6.5 (low)
- Cr 0.80 (WNL)
- Bili total 1.4 (high)
- Alk Phos 110 (WNL)
- Alb 3.1 (low)

- Amylase 250 U/L (high)
- Lipase 1150 U/L (high)
- Hgb 16.8 (high)

System review

- Heart: RRR
- Lungs: clear
- Extremities: no edema, cyanosis
- Chest: no rales or wheezing; normal breathing
- CV: Hx elevated cholesterol/triglycerides
- Abdomen: extremely tender abdomen, pain in epigastric and upper right quadrant, patient rates at a 10/10 pain level
- Neurologic: unremarkable, patient reports Hx of fibromyalgia

Assessment/Plan

1. Acute pancreatitis—We will admit the patient to the Medical floor and start IV fluids. D5 at 150 mL per hour. We will make her NPO. Seek CT scan of the abdomen to r/o cholelithiasis-induced pancreatitis vs chronic disease or from other etiologies. We will discontinue her oral medications and offer pain management IV.
2. Dyslipidemia—The patient has been on simvastatin. We will get a lipid panel with her next labs to assess this.
3. Depression—Patient has been on Zoloft and has been doing well on this.
4. Hypothyroidism—We will draw thyroid labs with next lab draw to assess current dose of levothyroxine.
5. Fibromyalgia—Not currently an issue.
6. Irritable bowel syndrome—Continues on Bentyl for both IBS and fibromyalgia. Not currently an issue but definitely needs to be monitored if patient requires surgery.
7. GERD—The patient is taking Prevacid. We will be able to provide this injection as the patient is NPO.

▶ Medication/Orders

Medication Orders	Amount	Route	Start Date
Levothyroxine	75 µg daily	HOLD	
Calcium/vitamin D-3	500 mg/400 IU	HOLD	
MVI with min	1 capsule daily	HOLD	
Simvastatin	20 mg daily	HOLD	
Dicyclomine	20 mg daily	HOLD	
Sertraline	25 mg daily	HOLD	
D5	150 mL/hour	IV	02/22/2017
Tramadol	50 mg every 6 hours Prn	IV	02/22/2017
Lansoprazole	30 mg—prn	Injectable	02/22/2017

Diet

NPO

Therapy Orders

R.D. consult for nutrition prn.
S.T. consult prn.

▸ Physician Progress Note 02/23/2017

Subjective

The patient states that she is still in pain but has improved. Obtained CT of the abdomen indicating a blocked common bile duct, which appears to be secondary to gallstones. We will collaborate with General Surgery to see if patient is a candidate for cholecystectomy and pursue that route. We will keep her NPO and hold oral meds. Continue with tramadol and IV fluids.

Objective

Vital signs

- Blood pressure: stable at 120/80
- O_2: 93%
- Weight: 167 lbs, up 2 lbs from admit weight

Abnormal lab values

- Sodium 136 (low)
- Albumin 3.0 (low)
- Calcium 7.9 (low)
- Bili 1.4
- ALT 59 (high)
- Alk Phos 132 (high)
- Almylase 230 (high)
- Lipase 550 (high)

Meds

Hold all oral meds, continue with IV fluids at 150 mL per hour, as well as IV tramadol.

Assessment

1. Cholelithiasis-induced pancreatitis with common bile duct obstruction.
2. Hyponatremia—We will change D5 to NaCl at 150 mL per hour. Check BMP and CMP daily.
3. Hypokalemia—We will provide a bolus of KCl of 80 mEq/L.
4. GERD—So far, patient has not needed lansoprazole. We will keep this medication prn.
5. Hyperlipidemia—Labs reviewed showing cholesterol 250 (high); LDL 135 (high); and triglycerides 300 (high). We will consider adding statin to her current regimen when she is able to take p.o. again. She may also need some dietary teaching.
6. Depression—No current issues.
7. Fibromyalgia—Not currently an issue.
8. IBS—Not currently an issue.

Plan

We will continue with IV fluids, changing to NaCl IV with a KCl bolus secondary to decreased electrolytes from fluid volume. We will continue patient NPO, in anticipation of cholecystectomy. Hopefully, after surgery, we will be able to advance her diet and get her to eat again. We will continue with IV pain control.

▸ Multidisciplinary Progress Notes

Nursing Progress Note 02/22/2017: 1015

BP 110/75, IV access to right arm infiltrated. Notified R.N. and IV restarted in left arm without complications. Patient c/o abdominal pain, starting tramadol IV per orders.

Nursing Progress Note
02/22/2017: 1300

Patient resting in bed in no acute distress. IV running at 150 mL per hour. Vitals taken. Patient reports no complaints at this time.

Nursing Progress Note
02/22/2017: 1700

Physician in to see patient and discussing possible surgery tomorrow for cholecystectomy. Patient remaining NPO; continues on IV fluids and IV pain management.

Nursing Progress Note
02/23/2017: 0930

Patient down to surgery for cholecystectomy.

Nursing Progress Note
02/23/2017: 1400

Patient returned from surgery. Remains NPO, but may have ice chips. Sleeping at this time. Following for orders. No intake so far p.o.

Nursing Progress Note
02/24/2017: 0800

Patient s/p surgery yesterday, diet advanced to clear liquids, poor appetite. She says her last "good" meal was about 6 days ago. Vitals taken, patient reports pain at 3 out of 10. BP taken at 125/70.

▸ Labs

CBC—02/22/2017

Test	Result	Units	Reference Ranges
WBC	8.5	×10³/uL	4.8–10.8
RBC	5.00	×10³/uL	4.10–6.70
Hemoglobin	16.8 (HI)	g/dL	12.5–16.0
Hematocrit	45.0	Percent	37.0–47.0
Erythrocyte MCV	90.4	fL	81.0–96.0
Erythrocyte MCH	36.0	pg	33.0–39.0
Erythrocyte MCHC	34.0	g/dL	32.0–36.0
RDW	16.0	Percent	13.0–18.0

(continues)

Test	Result	Units	Reference Ranges
MPV	8.6	fL	6.9–10.6
Platelet count	250	×10³/uL	130–400
Neutrophils (pct)	55.0	Percent	39.3–73.7
Neutrophils (ct)	3.0	×10³/uL	1.5–6.6
Lymphocytes (pct)	23.2	Percent	18.0–48.3
Lymphocytes (ct)	1.8	×10³/uL	1.1–2.9
Monocytes (pct)	5.1	Percent	4.4–12.7
Monocytes (ct)	0.3	×10³/uL	0.2–0.8
Eosinophils (pct)	0.9	Percent	0.6–7.3
Eosinophils (ct)	0.3	×10³/uL	0.0–0.4
Basophils (pct)	0.0	Percent	0.0–1.7
Basophils (ct)	0.0	×10³/uL	0.0–0.1

Lipid Panel—02/22/2017

Test	Result	Units	Reference Ranges
Total cholesterol	250 (HI)	mg/dL	<200 mg/dL
Triglyceride	300 (HI)	mg/dL	<150 mg/dL
HDL	48	mg/dL	>50 mg/dL—women
LDL	135 (HI)	mg/dL	<100 mg/dL
VLDL	33 (HI)	mg/dL	<30 mg/dL
Chol/HDL ratio	5.21 (HI)	Ratio	<5.0

CMP—02/22/2017

Test	Result	Units	Reference Ranges
Sodium	145	mmol/L	137–145
Potassium–serum	4.8	mmol/L	3.6–5.2
Chloride	109	mmol/L	100–110
Glucose	80	mg/dL	60–100
BUN	6.5 (LO)	mg/dL	7–17
Creatinine	0.80	mg/dL	0.52–1.04
Urea nitrogen/Cr ratio	8.1	Ratio	
GFR	>90	mL/minute	
Uric acid	6.0	mg/dL	2.5–6.2
Total protein	6.8	g/dL	6.5–8.1
Albumin	3.1 (LO)	g/dL	3.2–4.4
Globulin	3.69	g/dL	2.7–4.3
Albumin/globulin ratio	0.84	Ratio	
Calcium	7.8 (LO)	mg/dL	8.4–10.2
Bilirubin	1.4	mg/dL	0.2–1.3
ALT	50	U/L	9–52
AST	36	U/L	14–36
Alkaline phosphatase	130 (HI)	U/L	38–126
Amylase	250 (HI)	U/L	23–85
Lipase	1150 (HI)	U/L	0–160

(continues)

Test	Result	Units	Reference Ranges
Total bilirubin	1.4	mg/dL	0.3–1.9
TSH	1.35	mIU/L	0.32–5.00

CBC—02/23/2017

Test	Result	Units	Reference Ranges
WBC	10.0	×10³/uL	4.8–10.8
RBC	5.25	×10³/uL	4.10–6.70
Hemoglobin	13.0	g/dL	12.5–16.0
Hematocrit	40.0	Percent	37.0–47.0
Erythrocyte MCV	85.7	fL	81.0–96.0
Erythrocyte MCH	38.8	pg	33.0–39.0
Erythrocyte MCHC	34.5	g/dL	32.0–36.0
RDW	16.6	Percent	13.0–18.0
MPV	8.8	fL	6.9–10.6
Platelet count	200	×10³/uL	130–400
Neutrophils (pct)	58.0	Percent	39.3–73.7
Neutrophils (ct)	3.2	×10³/uL	1.5–6.6
Lymphocytes (pct)	29.2	Percent	18.0–48.3
Lymphocytes (ct)	2.0	×10³/uL	1.1–2.9
Monocytes (pct)	6.2	Percent	4.4–12.7
Monocytes (ct)	0.6	×10³/uL	0.2–0.8

Test	Result	Units	Reference Ranges
Eosinophils (pct)	0.9	Percent	0.6–7.3
Eosinophils (ct)	0.3	×10³/uL	0.0–0.4
Basophils (pct)	0.0	Percent	0.0–1.7
Basophils (ct)	0.0	×10³/uL	0.0–0.1

CMP—02/23/2017

Test	Result	Units	Reference Ranges
Sodium	136 (LO)	mmol/L	137–145
Potassium–serum	3.6 (LO)	mmol/L	3.6–5.2
Chloride	101	mmol/L	100–110
Glucose	85	mg/dL	60–100
BUN	7.7	mg/dL	7–17
Creatinine	1.00	mg/dL	0.52–1.04
Urea nitrogen/ Cr ratio	7.7	Ratio	
GFR	>90	mL/minute	
Uric acid	6.0	mg/dL	2.5–6.2
Total protein	6.7	g/dL	6.5–8.1
Albumin	3.0 (LO)	g/dL	3.2–4.4
Globulin	3.7	g/dL	2.7–4.3
Albumin/globulin ratio	0.81	Ratio	
Calcium	7.9 (LO)	mg/dL	8.4–10.2

(continues)

Test	Result	Units	Reference Ranges
ALT	59 (HI)	U/L	9–52
AST	35	U/L	14–36
Alkaline phosphatase	132 (HI)	U/L	38–126
Amylase	230 (HI)	U/L	23–85
Lipase	550 (HI)	U/L	0–160
Total bilirubin	1.8	mg/dL	0.3–1.9
TSH	1.35	mIU/L	0.32–5.00

▸ Nursing Intake and Output Queries

02/22/2017

Intake				
	0000–0800 hrs	0800–1600 hrs	1600–2400 hrs	24-hour total
IV/FL	1,508 mL	1,508 mL	1,508 mL	4,524 mL
PO	NPO	NPO	NPO	NPO
Total	**1,508 mL**	**1,508 mL**	**1,508 mL**	**4,524 mL**

Output				
	0000–0800 hrs	0800–1600 hrs	1600–2400 hrs	24-hour total
Urine	250 mL	300 mL	300 mL	850 mL
Urine	400 mL	180 mL	300 mL	880 mL
BM				
Total	**650 mL**	**480 mL**	**600 mL**	**1,730 mL**

24-hour total fluid balance: 2,794 mL.

02/23/2017

Intake				
	0000–0800 hrs	0800–1600 hrs	1600–2400 hrs	24-hour total
IV/FL	1,508 mL	1,508 mL	1,508 mL	4,524 mL
PO	NPO	NPO	NPO	NPO
Total	**1,508 mL**	**1,508 mL**	**1,508 mL**	**4,524 mL**

Output				
	0000–0800 hrs	0800–1600 hrs	1600–2400 hrs	24-hour total
Urine	275 mL	310 mL	350 mL	935 mL
Urine	200 mL	200 mL	300 mL	700 mL
BM				
Total	**475 mL**	**510 mL**	**650 mL**	**1,635 mL**

24-hour total fluid balance: 2,889 mL.

02/24/2017

Intake				
	0000–0800 hrs	0800–1600 hrs	1600–2400 hrs	24-hour total
IV/FL	1,508 mL			
PO	120 mL			
Total	**1,628 mL**			

Output				
	0000–0800 hrs	0800–1600 hrs	1600–2400 hrs	24-hour total
Urine	120 mL			
Urine	120 mL			
BM				
Total	**240 mL**			

Meal Record

	Breakfast	Snack	Lunch	Snack	Dinner	Snack	24-hour Total
02/22/2017	NPO		NPO		NPO		NPO
02/23/2017	NPO		NPO		NPO		NPO
02/24/2017	120 mL						

Weight Log

	02/22/2017	02/23/2017	02/24/2017	02/25/2017
Method	**Bed Scale**	**Bed Scale**	**Bed Scale**	
Weight (lbs)	165	167	169	
Weight (kg)	75	75.9	76.3	
Height (in)	65			

▶ Resources

Evidenced-based practice guidelines, protocols, or algorithms used in creating scenarios include the following. Students may wish to review these resources in preparation for the simulation scenario.

- Kane and Prelack. *Advanced Medical Nutrition Therapy*. Jones & Bartlett Learning: Burlington, 2018.
- Academy of Nutrition and Dietetics. Evidence Based Practice Guidelines.
- Academy of Nutrition and Dietetics. Nutrition Care Manual.
- Academy of Nutrition and Dietetics. Academy of Nutrition and Dietetics Health Informatics Infrastructure (ANDHII). www.andhii.org/info.

- Safaii-Waite. *Medical Nutrition Therapy Simulations*. Online module: Acute pancreatitis. Jones & Bartlett Learning: Burlington, 2017.

▶ Key Words

Amylase
Cholelithiasis
Common Bile Duct
Gallstones
Infiltrated
Lipase
Pancreatitis
Tramadol

SIMULATION SCENARIO:

Renal Failure

LEARNING OBJECTIVES

- Identify different nutrition interventions for renal failure and how to select the appropriate intervention
- Be able to identify the recommended nutrition therapy for patients with end-stage renal disease
- Estimate protein, calories, and fluid needs for a patient with renal failure who is on hemodialysis; adjust IBW for a below-the-knee amputation

▶ Student and Instructor Preparation

- Read chapter and lecture notes on medical nutrition therapy for renal failure
- Understand national MNT guidelines for end-stage renal-disease, including malnutrition, stress, unhealthy eating habits, smoking, alcohol consumption, diabetes, age, impaired immunity, and other chronic diseases, such as hypertension
- Review Evidence Based Library of the Academy of Nutrition and Dietetics
- Review equations for estimation of energy, protein needs, and fluid needs for a patient with chronic renal failure receiving hemodialysis
- Practice online simulation module for renal failure

▶ Lab Set Up

Patient: Abe Richman

Patient characteristics: The patient is a 60-year-old male who has been on hemodialysis for 8 years. He is a retired history teacher and lives at home with his spouse, who is his primary caregiver. He has unfortunately had a left-leg-below-the-knee amputation R/T diabetic neuropathy. He and his spouse have two children who both live close and, at times, help to prepare meals and assist with household chores. His family is very important to him. He often suffers from bouts of major depression and anxiety, but the support of his family helps him through difficult times.

Environment/setting/location: Hospital in-patient setting; patient hospital room.

Lab staff needed on day of simulation: Preceptor/evaluator (1) or patient (1) (can be another preceptor/instructor, sim man, another student or actor). Preferable to have one actor for patient's spouse and two additional actors for patient's adult children.

Equipment, supplies, and prop list: Hospital room, bed, privacy curtain, bedside table, water mug, pillow, blanket, three additional folding chairs at bedside. Optional: snack on bedside table, such as diet soda.

▶ Clinical Case Information

Subjective

Abe is a 60-year-old male on hemodialysis with an amputation to the left lower leg below the knee, which was performed 1 year ago. This was related to uncontrolled diabetes, resulting in severe diabetic neuropathy and an infection which, despite multiple attempts to treat, did not resolve. He is treated by Dr. Shoemaker for hemodialysis, whom he has been seeing for nearly 8 years. He is here due to a failed right arm AV fistula, which is being replaced today. He has tremendous family support. His spouse is his primary caregiver, and both of his children are involved in assisting the patient when his wife needs to be relieved. He is a retired history teacher. Despite multiple attempts to educate the patient, the dialysis center reports that this patient has had a difficult time limiting milk products in his diet and giving up diet soda. He also has severe depressive episodes at

times and uses food as a means of coping with this. His wife says they try to follow the diet outlined by the dialysis R.D., but state that Abe has had a poor appetite and she would rather he eat something than nothing at all. Physical assessment reveals subcutaneous fat loss to temporal, clavicle, and scapular regions.

Objective
Vital signs

- Blood pressure: 123/78
- Temperature: 98°F
- O_2: 96% on room air
- Weight: 218 lbs
- Height: 5'8"
- UBW: ~250 lbs
- Weight loss of 30 lbs × 1 year

Meds

- Lantus insulin 60 units daily
- Humalog 20 units per meal
- Lisinopril 40 mg/daily
- Simvastatin 20 mg/day
- Metoprolol 100 mg daily
- Sensipar 120 mg/day
- Fish oil 1,000 mg capsule twice daily
- Nephrovite daily
- Vitamin D-3 2,000 IU daily
- Prednisone 10 mg daily with food
- Tums, two tablets t.i.d. with meals

System review

- Heart: unremarkable, no current problems.
- Lungs: clear, no rattles, wheezing, or crackles.
- Extremities: Patient has had left lower extremity below-the-knee amputation.
- CV: Patient with chronic hypertension. Edema—trace to right lower extremity. No fluid retention noted to hands or trunk.
- Abdomen: nontender, no organomegaly; obese.

- Neurologic: Patient c/o shooting pain down through right lower leg at times; tingling pain in hands. No lightheadedness, dizziness.

PMHx

- HTN
- Hyperparathyroidism secondary to CKD
- Anemia of chronic disease
- ESRD (Stage 5)
- Arthritis
- Vitamin D deficiency
- Hyperlipidemia
- Type 2 diabetes mellitus

Family Hx

Patient's father died from a heart attack at age 76. Patient's mother is alive and has diabetes and heart disease. Patient is the youngest of four siblings, one deceased brother who died in a MVA; three siblings living; two with diabetes, HTN, and one with rheumatoid arthritis.

Social Hx

Patient has a Hx of mild ETOH use. He has never smoked or used recreational drugs.

Surgical Hx

Cholecystectomy at age 25; Right ankle tendon repair at age 38; Rt AV fistula placement 7.5 years ago. Left lower extremity below-the-knee amputation 1 year ago.

Abnormal lab values

- Hgb 12.0 (low)
- Hct 35.0 (low)
- MCV 98.9 (high)
- Na$^+$ 132 (low)
- K$^+$ 3.2 (low)
- Cl 96 (low)
- Glucose 155 (high)
- BUN 101 (high)

- Cr 6.00 (high)
- Phosphatase 6.5 (high)

Allergies

Walnuts, latex

Assessment

1. Hemodialysis patient with a failed right sided AV fistula. Here for replacement.
2. Type 2 diabetes mellitus, with Hx of uncontrolled blood sugars resulting in kidney failure. Will continue to limit carbohydrates to 75 grams per meal.
3. Hyperparathyroidism—Secondary to CKD. Continue sensipar. Not currently an issue.
4. Hypertension—Patient is on metoprolol 100 mg daily. Will continue same dosage.
5. Vitamin D deficiency—Continue with supplemental vitamin D.
6. Hyperlipidemia—The patient is on simvastatin 20 mg daily.
7. Arthritis—The patient is taking prednisone daily; no current issues with this.
8. Left lower extremity below-the-knee amputation 1 year ago related to diabetic neuropathy and multiple failed attempts at treating infectious process of this lower limb.

Plan

We will contact Surgery for consultation involving a failed right-sided AV fistula. Will consult Dr. Meyer for assistance in getting the patient dialyzed and seek placement of a central venous catheter to do so as he will need this access for the next couple of months while his fistula heals. We will cover him with a broad-spectrum IV antibiotic prophylaxis. We will work with interdisciplinary therapies as needed. His diet will address his diabetes and renal compromise. Will seek consult from Clinical Nutrition to address diet compliance with patient, as well as assist in helping with his appetite.

▶ Physician Progress Note 08/02/2017

Subjective

Patient reports he is feeling better today. A new fistula was placed on the left side (arm) and patient tolerated the procedure well. He had dialysis this morning and is more alert and states his appetite is a little better; he has tolerated full liquid s/p surgery and we will continue to advance his diet today. Fistula shows no signs of infection and appears to be healing well. We will get the patient up and moving this morning since he has finished and tolerated his dialysis procedure without hypotensive episodes.

Objective

Vital signs

- Blood pressure: stable at 135/87
- O_2: 92% on room air
- Weight: 209 lbs
- Predialysis weight 8 years ago 268 lbs; he has steadily lost weight since starting dialysis, but most recently, 20 lbs in 1 year

Abnormal lab values

- Hct 36.6 (low)
- MCV 99.0 (high)
- Cl 99 (low)
- Glucose 137 (high)
- BUN 96 (high)
- Cr 4.75 (high)
- Phosphatase 6.00 (high)

Meds

- Lantus insulin 60 units daily
- Humalog 20 units per meal
- Lisinopril 40 mg/daily
- Simvastatin 20 mg/day
- Metroprolol 100 mg daily
- Sensipar 120 mg daily
- Nephrovite daily
- Vitamin D-3 2,000 IU daily
- Tums, two tabs t.i.d. with meals
- Prednisone 10 mg daily with food
- IV Vancomycin

Allergies

Walnuts, latex

Assessment

1. ESRD—Patient is receiving hemodialysis via central venous access for the next couple of months until left AV fistula heals. Will collaborate with Nursing as patient will need to learn how to keep this access clean and how to watch for infection and other problems. He may also need education regarding his diet, although he has had this before. He may just lack motivation to limit high phosphorus foods.
2. Type 2 diabetes mellitus, uncontrolled—We will continue with Lantus and sliding scale insulin, as ordered. The patient's capillary glucose values have shown some improvement with this.
3. Hypercholesterolemia—Will continue with simvastatin.
4. Hyperparathyroid—No current issues. Continue with sensipar.
5. Weight loss and poor appetite—The patient reports a weight loss of 20 lbs in the past year related to poor appetite. We will certainly consult Nutrition to help with this.

$$1,775.5$$

$$(10 \cdot 99.1) + 6.25(172.72) - 300 + 5$$
$$991 + 1,079.5 \qquad \times 1.3$$

▶ Medication/Orders

Medication Orders	Amount	Route	Start Date
Metoprolol	100 mg daily	p.o.	08/01/2017
Lisinopril	40 mg daily	p.o.	08/01/2017
Sensipar	120 mg daily	p.o.	08/01/2017
Simvastatin	20 mg/day	p.o.	08/01/2017
Nephrovite	1 cap daily	p.o.	08/01/2017
Calcium carbonate (Tums)	2 cap t.i.d. w/meals	p.o.	08/01/2017
Vitamin D-3 2,000 IU daily	1 cap daily	p.o.	08/01/2017
Acetaminophen	325 mg q 6 hrs prn	p.o.	08/01/2017
Acetaminophen	325 mg q 6 hrs prn	IV	08/01/2017
Ondansetron	4–8 mg q 6 hrs prn	p.o.	08/01/2017
Ondansetron	4–8 mg q 6 hrs prn	IV	08/01/2017
Simethicone	80 mg q 2 hrs prn	p.o.	08/01/2017
Lantus insulin	60 units q HS	IM	08/01/2017
Sliding Scale Humalog	(Refer to moderate dose SS policy)		08/01/2017
NaCl 0.45%	50 mL q 6 hrs		
Add Vancomycin	1250 mg	One-time dose	08/01/2017
NaCl 0.45%	50 mL q 6 hrs		
Add piperacillin/tazobactam	2.25 g q 6 hrs	IV	08/01/2017

Diet

NPO	0700 08/01/2017
Clear Liquids	1630 08/01/2017
Full liquids—Renal 80 g protein,	
75 g consistent carbohydrate (1 g Phos,	
2 gm K$^+$, 2 gm Na$^+$)	0700 08/02/2017

Therapy Orders
08/01/2017

R.D. consult for nutrition and diet needs prn.
S.T. consult prn.
Social Services consult with discharge planning, as needed.

▶ Multidisciplinary Progress Notes

Nursing Progress Note
08/01/2017: 1000

Patient is NPO, resting in bed s/p left AV fistula placement and central venous catheter placement. Patient is to receive hemodialysis today.

Nursing Progress Note
08/01/2017: 1300

Patient continues NPO, awaiting order for diet advancement as he has shown good tolerance of dialysis procedure. Patience reports no nausea or vomiting. States that appetite is fair. Patient's family in room and at bedside. Patient declined to walk with P.T.

Nursing Progress Note
08/01/2017: 1530

MD wrote for diet to advance to clear liquids. Patient accepted grape juice. No nausea or vomiting. Family still in patient's room, asking to speak with physician regarding recovery and care of new access site. Family expresses concerns about inability to care for patient at home.

Nursing Progress Note
08/02/2017: 0700

Order for diet advance to renal diet with 75 g carbohydrates per meal. Notified patient of ordering system so he can order breakfast. Patient's spouse says she will order for him. Patient reports that he is not hungry and asked for a chocolate Boost drink. Patient drank Boost for breakfast. BG 179 mg/dL. Insulin given according to orders.

Nursing Progress Note
08/02/2017: 1125

Patient up to restroom with 180 mL urine output. Fistula site clean and without signs or symptoms of infection. Patient ate two saltine crackers and drank apple juice at snack time. Patient's wife brought in a snickers bar and tried to get him to eat it. She said he will eat this if he is not feeling well. Encouraged family to order meals from the menu provided.

Social Services Progress Note
08/02/2017: 1330

Visited with family regarding concerns for caring for patient at home while fistula is healing. They are considering placing patient for short-term stay. Will collaborate with discharge planning and continue to visit with family regarding their wishes.

▶ Labs

CBC—08/01/2017

Test	Result	Units	Reference Ranges
WBC	7.8	×10³/uL	4.8–10.8
RBC	6.20	×10³/uL	4.10–6.70
Hemoglobin	12.0 (LO)	g/dL	12.5–16.0
Hematocrit	35.0 (LO)	Percent	37.0–47.0
Erythrocyte MCV	98.9 (HI)	fL	81.0–96.0
Erythrocyte MCH	35.5	pg	33.0–39.0
Erythrocyte MCHC	34.5	g/dL	32.0–36.0
RDW	13.8	Percent	13.0–18.0
MPV	7.0	fL	6.9–10.6
Platelet count	350	×10³/uL	130–400
Neutrophils (pct)	70.3	Percent	39.3–73.7
Neutrophils (ct)	6.0	×10³/uL	1.5–6.6
Lymphocytes (pct)	55.5	Percent	18.0–48.3
Lymphocytes (ct)	2.0	×10³/uL	1.1–2.9
Monocytes (pct)	4.4	Percent	4.4–12.7
Monocytes (ct)	0.2	×10³/uL	0.2–0.8
Eosinophils (pct)	2.0	Percent	0.6–7.3
Eosinophils (ct)	0.0	×10³/uL	0.0–0.4
Basophils (pct)	0.3	Percent	0.0–1.7
Basophils (ct)	0.0	×10³/uL	0.0–0.1

CMP—08/01/2017

would it be more important to have them stick to kidney diet or to decrease weight/lipids

Test	Result	Units	Reference Ranges
Sodium	132 (LO)	mmol/L	137–145
Potassium–serum	3.2 (LO)	mmol/L	3.6–5.2
Chloride	96 (LO)	mmol/L	100–110
Glucose	155 (HI)	mg/dL	60–100
BUN	101 (HI)	mg/dL	7–17
Creatinine	6.00 (HI)	mg/dL	0.52–1.04
Urea nitrogen/ Cr ratio	20.2	Ratio	
GFR	12 (LO)	mL/minute	
Phosphatase	6.5 (HI)	mg/dL	2.4–4.1
Uric acid	5.6	mg/dL	2.5–6.2
Total protein	6.4 (LO)	g/dL	6.5–8.1
Albumin	3.0 (LO)	g/dL	3.2–4.4
Globulin	3.4	g/dL	2.7–4.3
Albumin/globulin ratio	0.88	Ratio	
Calcium	8.8	mg/dL	8.4–10.2
Bilirubin	1.0	mg/dL	0.2–1.3
ALT	45	U/L	9-52
AST	30	U/L	14–36
Alkaline phosphatase	96	U/L	38–126
TSH	3.00	mIU/L	0.32–5.00

CBC—08/02/2017

Test	Result	Units	Reference Ranges
WBC	7.0	×10³/uL	4.8–10.8
RBC	6.50	×10³/uL	4.10–6.70
Hemoglobin	12.9	g/dL	12.5–16.0
Hematocrit	36.6 (LO)	Percent	37.0–47.0
Erythrocyte MCV	99.0 (HI)	fL	81.0–96.0
Erythrocyte MCH	35.0	pg	33.0–39.0
Erythrocyte MCHC	35.5	g/dL	32.0–36.0
RDW	14.0	Percent	13.0–18.0
MPV	7.0	fL	6.9–10.6
Platelet count	280	×10³/uL	130–400
Neutrophils (pct)	65.0	Percent	39.3–73.7
Neutrophils (ct)	6.0	×10³/uL	1.5–6.6
Lymphocytes (pct)	45.0	Percent	18.0–48.3
Lymphocytes (ct)	2.3	×10³/uL	1.1–2.9
Monocytes (pct)	4.9	Percent	4.4–12.7
Monocytes (ct)	0.5	×10³/uL	0.2–0.8
Eosinophils (pct)	3.5	Percent	0.6–7.3
Eosinophils (ct)	0.0	×10³/uL	0.0–0.4
Basophils (pct)	0.1	Percent	0.0–1.7
Basophils (ct)	0.0	×10³/uL	0.0–0.1

CMP—08/02/2017

Test	Result	Units	Reference Ranges
Sodium	138	mmol/L	137–145
Potassium–serum	4.8	mmol/L	3.6–5.2
Chloride	99 (LO)	mmol/L	100–110
Glucose	137 (HI)	mg/dL	60–100
BUN	96 (HI)	mg/dL	7–17
Creatinine	5.75	mg/dL	0.52–1.04
Urea nitrogen/Cr ratio	20.2	Ratio	
GFR	12.5 (LO)	mL/minute	
Phosphatase	6.2 (HI)	mg/dL	2.4–4.1
Uric acid	4.8	mg/dL	2.5–6.2
Total protein	6.9	g/dL	6.5–8.1
Albumin	3.2 (LO)	g/dL	3.2–4.4
Globulin	3.7	g/dL	2.7–4.3
Albumin/globulin ratio	0.86	Ratio	
Calcium	9.0	mg/dL	8.4–10.2
Bilirubin	1.0	mg/dL	0.2–1.3
ALT	40	U/L	9–52
AST	35	U/L	14–36
Alkaline phosphatase	90	U/L	38–126

▶ Nursing Intake and Output Queries

08/01/2017

Intake				
	0000–0800 hrs	0800–1600 hrs	1600–2400 hrs	24-hour total
IV/FL		50 mL	50 mL	100 mL
PO		NPO	360 mL	360 mL
Total		**50 mL**	**410 mL**	**460 mL**

Output				
	0000–0800 hrs	0800–1600 hrs	1600–2400 hrs	24-hour total
Urine	50 mL		50 mL	100 mL
BM	Large			
Dialysis		2,600 mL		2,600 mL
Total	**50 mL**	**2,600 mL**	**50 mL**	**2,700 mL**

24-hour total fluid balance: −2,240 mL.

08/02/2017

Intake				
	0000–0800 hrs	0800–1600 hrs	1600–2400 hrs	24-hour total
IV/FL	50 mL	50 mL		
PO	300 mL	400 mL		
PO	120 mL			
Total	**470 mL**	**450 mL**		

Output				
	0000–0800 hrs	0800–1600 hrs	1600–2400 hrs	24-hour total
Urine	50 mL	180 mL		
BM				
Total	**50 mL**	**180 mL**		

Meal Record

	Breakfast	Snack	Lunch	Snack	Dinner	Snack	24-hour Total
08/01/2017	NPO		NPO		200 mL	100%	400 mL
08/02/2017	300 mL	120	400 mL				820 mL

Weight Log

	08/01/2017	08/02/2017	08/03/2017	08/04/2017
Method	**Bed Scale**	**Bed Scale**		
Weight (lbs)	218	209		
Weight (kg)	99.0	95.0		
Height (in)	68			

▶ Capillary Glucose Values

08/01/2017

0800	1200	1730	2200
160	197	175	130
8 units Humalog	10 units Humalog	9 units Humalog	

08/02/2017

0800	1200	1730	2200
145	150		
5 units Humalog	5 units Humalog		

▶ Resources

Evidenced-based practice guidelines, protocols, or algorithms used in creating scenarios include the following. Students may wish to review these resources in preparation for the simulation scenario.

- Kane and Prelack. *Advanced Medical Nutrition Therapy.* Jones & Bartlett Learning: Burlington, 2018.
- Academy of Nutrition and Dietetics. Evidence Based Practice Guidelines.
- Academy of Nutrition and Dietetics. Nutrition Care Manual.
- Academy of Nutrition and Dietetics. Academy of Nutrition and Dietetics Health Informatics Infrastructure (ANDHII). https://www.andhii.org/info/.
- Safaii-Waite. *Medical Nutrition Therapy Simulations.* Online module: Renal failure. Jones & Bartlett Learning: Burlington, 2017.

▶ Key Words

Amputation R/T
End-stage renal disease
Fistula
Hemodialysis
Hyperparathyroidism
Levothyroxine
Metoprolol
Renal failure
Simvastatin

SIMULATION SCENARIO:

Wound Care

LEARNING OBJECTIVES

- Identify several different nutrition interventions that could help in wound healing and how to select the appropriate intervention
- Be able to identify the recommended nutrition therapy for wound healing
- Estimate appropriate protein, calories, and fluid needs for patient based on recommended calculations for estimated needs

▶ Student and Instructor Preparation

- Read chapter and lecture notes on MNT for wound healing
- Understand national MNT guidelines for helping to heal and maintain skin integrity, including: malnutrition, stress, unhealthy eating habits, smoking, alcohol consumption, diabetes, age, impaired immunity, and chronic disease
- Review Evidence Based Library of the Academy of Nutrition and Dietetics
- Review stages of wound healing, including: inflammatory phase, proliferative phase, and remodeling phase
- Review equations for estimation of calorie, protein, and fluid needs for wound patient
- Practice online decision-tree module for wound care

▶ Lab Set Up

Patient: J.D.

Patient characteristics: J.D. is a 65-year-old male who is a retired farmer. He is a pleasant person and likes to visit with others. He is physically active on the farm that he grew up on (and still lives). He is easy to get along with and willing to learn new information. Patient is eating a late lunch during R.D.'s visit.

Environment/setting/location: Patient hospital room, lights on and window curtain open; afternoon visit.

Lab staff needed on day of simulation: Preceptor/evaluator (1) and patient (1) (can be another preceptor/instructor, sim man, another student or actor).

Equipment, supplies, and prop list: Hospital room, bed, food tray, bedside table, water mug on tray next to bed.

▶ Clinical Case Information (06/08/2017)

Subjective

J.D. is a 67-year-old retired farmer/rancher who has been known to this physician for many years. Two weeks ago, he was seen by myself, Dr. Smith, for cough, fever, and overall malaise. He was diagnosed with bronchitis and sent home on ABX therapy for 5 days. He continued to worsen over the past week after he finished the ABX and reported that he just had not been able to get out of bed. The patient claims that he is incontinent of bladder at times, which certainly does not help, as he has been mostly bedridden for the past week. He also reports no interest in eating. He has been sipping coffee and eating toast, but his appetite is very poor and he has eaten very little of anything else. He comes in for evaluation today, brought in by his neighbor, for increased weakness, worsening tightness in chest, fever spikes, and severe weakness.

Objective

Vital signs

- Blood pressure: 145/89
- Temperature: 99.8°F
- Heart rate 87 bpm, respiration 20 per minute
- O_2: saturation 90% on 2 liters O_2

System review

- HEENT/neck: unremarkable, and no tenderness.
- Chest: Severe rattles, crackles. Some noted wheezing.
- Cardiovascular: Regular rate and rhythm.
- Abdomen: Soft, nontender, with active bowel sounds.
- Extremities: No edema.
- Skin: Exam reveals skin breakdown to buttocks, stage 3.
- Neurologic: Intact, no concerns.

Objective

Vital signs

- Patient's weight is 145 lbs
- Height: 5'7"
- Past medical Hx indicates weight 6 months ago was 151 lbs

Abnormal lab values and x-ray

- Na^+ 131 (low)
- K^+ 3.0 (low)
- Glucose 111 (high)
- CRP 7.9 (high)
- BUN 27 (high)
- Cr 2.01 (high)
- Total protein 6.0 (low)
- Albumin 2.8 (low)
- Ca^{++} 8.0 (low)
- Hgb 10.1 (low)
- Hct 30.2 (low)
- X-ray reveals left lower lobe infiltrate consistent with pneumonia
- WBC 14.4 (high)

PMHx

COPD, HTN, GERD, depression, BPH, hyperlipidemia

Social Hx

Smoker with ½ pack a day Hx, patient quit smoking 10 years ago. He lives alone, as his spouse died 10 years ago from cancer.

Family Hx

Patient's father died at age 87 from a heart attack. His mother died at age 90 from unknown illness. Patient's siblings are still alive, one brother with DM, and a sister with Hx of breast cancer.

Meds

- Aspirin 81 mg daily
- HCTZ
- Avodart
- Elavil
- Prilosec
- Spiriva inhaler

Assessment/Plan

1. Sepsis R/T acute on chronic hypoxic respiratory failure from COPD, likely pneumonia. Continue Spiriva and IV ABX.
2. Left lower-lobe pneumonia. Likely multiorganism per x-ray; cultures pending. Will cover at this point with a combination of trimethoprim and sulfamethoxazole. Add steroids, if needed based on outcomes.
3. GERD—Continue Prilosec.
4. Depression—Patient reports this is not an issue. Continue with Elavil.
5. BPH—Continue with Avodart.
6. HTN—Continue with HCTZ. We may need to look at other meds in conjunction with this if the patient's blood pressure continues to elevate. D/C aspirin.
7. Will consult with Dr. Jones regarding wound care as the patient has developed a pressure area that has progressed to stage 3.
8. Start daily MVI with minerals.
9. Malnutrition R/T poor intake >7 days with weight loss.
10. CKD stage 3—We will continue to manage patient's blood pressure. No indications of proteinuria.

▶ Medication/Orders

Medication Orders	Amount	Route	Start Date
Prilosec	20 mg daily	p.o.	06/06/2017
Sulfamethoxazole/trimethoprim	200 mg/30 mg q 8 hours	IV	06/06/2017
D5	100 mL/hour	IV	06/06/2017
Elavil	10 mg q 8 hours; 20 mg at bedtime	p.o.	06/06/2017
MVI with minerals	1 cap daily	p.o.	06/06/2017
Avodart	0.5 mg daily	p.o.	06/06/2017
Acetaminophen	325 mg q 8 hours prn	p.o.	

(continues)

Medication Orders	Amount	Route	Start Date
Ondansetron	4–8 mg q 6 hrs prn	p.o.	06/06/2017
Simethicone	80 mg q 2 hrs prn	p.o.	06/06/2017
HCTZ	50 mg daily	p.o.	06/06/2017

Diet

Regular   06/06/2017

Therapy Orders
06/07/2017

P.T. to ambulate 2× to 3× daily, work with strengthening and balance.
R.D. consult as needed for nutrition and intake.
S.T. consult prn.
Social Services consult with discharge planning for possible ECF placement for rehabilitation.

▸ Interdisciplinary Progress Notes

Social Services Progress Note
06/08/2017

Patient is a 67-year-old male who lives alone as his wife passed away 10 years ago due to cancer. He is usually physically active, but since he got sick, he has been bedridden R/T weakness. He used to smoke but doesn't anymore. Assessed needs during interview with patient. He likes to talk about his life on his farm. His closest neighbor is 1 mile away from him and patient reports that neighbor could check on him occasionally when he goes home. Patient may be a candidate for ECF for short-term stay after hospitalization for strengthening, if his weakness continues. Patient quit smoking 10 years ago without relapse.

Nursing Progress Note
06/08/2017: 0800

Skin assessment completed, note stage 3 pressure area to bilateral buttocks. Patient says he was bedridden for a week. Covered with Tegaderm and encouraged patient to turn often.

Physical Therapy Progress Note
06/08/2017: 0915

Orders for ambulating patient 2× to 3× daily. Patient continues to be weak and relies on therapy for support. Will continue to work with patient on strengthening and balance. May benefit from ECF short stay due to weakness.

Wound Progress Note
06/08/2017: 1640

Skin assessment completed and in agreement with R.N. note 06/08/2017 at 0800. Continue to cover, no concerns with wound bed that would impede healing. Reassessment reveals that wound has progressed to Stage 3. Continue to cover. Encourage patient to turn every 2 hours, as recently, he has not been following nursing recommendations.

Nursing Assistant
06/08/2017: 1810

Blood pressure 145/89; patient is sitting up in bed, watching T.V. Continues to ask C.N.A. to find call light and telephone for him. Patient is occasionally incontinent of bladder.

▶ Labs

CBC—06/07/2017

Test	Results	Units	Reference Ranges
WBC	14.4 (HI)	×10³/uL	4.8–10.8
RBC	6.5	×10³/uL	4.10–6.70
Hemoglobin	10.1 (LO)	g/dL	12.5–16.0
Hematocrit	30.2 (LO)	Percent	37.0–47.0
Erythrocyte MCV	94.6	fL	81.0–96.0
Erythrocyte MCH	32.4 (LO)	pg	33.0–39.0
Erythrocyte MCHC	34.2	g/dL	32.0–36.0
RDW	15.7	Percent	13.0–18.0
MPV	7.7	fL	6.9–10.6
Platelet count	344	×10³/uL	130–400
Neutrophils (pct)	45.5	Percent	39.3–73.7
Neutrophils (ct)	5.5	×10³/uL	1.5–6.6
Lymphocytes (pct)	20.8	Percent	18.0–48.3
Lymphocytes (ct)	2.0	×10³/uL	1.1–2.9
Monocytes (pct)	6.8	Percent	4.4–12.7
Monocytes (ct)	0.5	×10³/uL	0.2–0.8
Eosinophils (pct)	4.3	Percent	0.6–7.3
Eosinophils (ct)	0.1	×10³/uL	0.0–0.4
Basophils (pct)	0.9	Percent	0.0–1.7
Basophils (ct)	0.0	×10³/uL	0.0–0.1

CMP—06/07/2017

Test	Results	Units	Reference Ranges
Sodium	131 (LO)	mmol/L	137–145
Potassium–serum	3.0 (LO)	mmol/L	3.6–5.2
Chloride–serum	98 (LO)	mmol/L	100–110
Glucose	111 (HI)	mg/dL	60–100
BUN	27 (HI)	mg/dL	7–17
Creatinine	2.01 (HI)	mg/dL	0.52–1.04
Urea nitrogen/Cr ratio	13.4	Ratio	
GFR	34	mL/min	
Uric acid	5.5	mg/dL	2.5–6.2
Total protein	6.0 (LO)	g/dL	6.5–8.1
Albumin	2.8 (LO)	g/dL	3.2–4.4
Globulin	3.3	g/dL	2.7–4.3
Albumin/globulin ratio	0.87	Ratio	
Calcium	8.0 (LO)	mg/dL	8.4–10.2
Bilirubin	0.9	mg/dL .	0.2–1.3
ALT	33	U/L	9–52
AST	24	U/L	14–36
Alkaline phosphatase	87	U/L	38–126
CRP	7.9 (HI)	mg/L	<1.0 mg/L

▶ Nursing Intake and Output Queries

06/07/2017

Intake				
	0000–0800 hrs	0800–1600 hrs	1600–2400 hrs	24-hour total
IV/FL	800 mL	800 mL	800 mL	2,400 mL
PO	180 mL	200 mL	240 mL	620 mL
PO	50 mL	100 mL	240 mL	390 mL
Total	**1,030 mL**	**1,100 mL**	**1,280 mL**	**3,410 mL**

Output				
	0000–0800 hrs	0800–1600 hrs	1600–2400 hrs	24-hour total
Urine	300 mL	180 mL	240 mL	720 mL
Urine	220 mL	120 mL	200 mL	540 mL
BM	0			0
Total	**520 mL**	**300 mL**	**440 mL**	**1,260 mL**

24-hour total fluid balance: 2,150 mL.

Meal Record

	Breakfast	Snack	Lunch	Snack	Dinner	Snack	24-hour Total
06/07/2017	10%		15%		30%		18.3%
06/08/2017	30%						

Weight Log

	06/07/2017	06/08/2017		
Method	Bed Scale	Bed Scale		
Weight (lbs)	143	145		
Weight (kg)	65	65.9		
Height (in)	67			

▶ Resources

Evidenced-based practice guidelines, protocols, or algorithms used in creating scenarios include the following. Students may wish to review these resources in preparation for the simulation scenario.

- Kane and Prelack. *Advanced Medical Nutrition Therapy.* Jones & Bartlett Learning: Burlington, 2018.
- Academy of Nutrition and Dietetics. Evidence Based Practice Guidelines.
- Academy of Nutrition and Dietetics. Nutrition Care Manual.
- Academy of Nutrition and Dietetics. Academy of Nutrition and Dietetics Health Informatics Infrastructure (ANDHII). https://www.andhii.org/info/.

- Safaii-Waite. *Medical Nutrition Therapy Simulations.* Online module: Wound care. Jones & Bartlett Learning: Burlington, 2017.

▶ Key Words

ABX therapy
BPH
COPD
GERD
HTN
Hyperlipidemia
Tegaderm
Ulcer Stage 1; Stage 2; Stage 3; Stage 4

Glossary

A

Abdominal paracentesis A simple in-office procedure in which a needle is inserted into the peritoneal cavity and ascetic fluid is removed.

ABX therapy Antibiotics therapy

Acidosis An overproduction of acid in the blood or an excessive loss of bicarbonate from the blood (metabolic acidosis) or by a buildup of carbon dioxide in the blood that results from poor lung function or depressed breathing (respiratory acidosis).

Ammonia A pungent, colorless, gaseous alkaline compound of nitrogen and hydrogen (NH_3), which is very soluble in water and can easily be condensed to a liquid by cold and pressure.

Amputation R/T The removal of a limb related to (R/T) trauma, medical illness, or surgery.

Amylase Enzymes (as amylopsin) that catalyze the hydrolysis of starch and glycogen or their intermediate hydrolysis products.

Anemic A condition characterized by a deficiency of oxygen in body tissues, resulting from a decrease in the number of erythrocytes in the blood or in the amount of hemoglobin.

Aphasia Loss or impairment of the power to use or comprehend words, usually resulting from brain damage, which makes it hard to read, write, or communicate.

Arthroplasty The operative formation or restoration of a joint.

Autoimmune disease One of a large group of diseases characterized by the subversion or alteration of the function of the immune system of the body.

B

BPH Benign prostatic hyperplasia, benign prostatic hypertrophy.

Bronchitis An inflammation of the air passages between the nose and the lungs, including the windpipe or trachea and the larger air tubes of the lung that bring air in from the trachea (bronchi). Bronchitis can either be of brief duration (acute) or have a long course (chronic). It can be caused by a viral or a bacterial infection.

Budesonide A glucocorticoid anti-inflammatory administered by inhalation.

C

Cancer A malignant tumor that expands locally by invasion and systemically by metastasis.

Celiac disease (Gluten-sensitive enteropathy) A chronic, hereditary intestinal disorder in which an inability to absorb the gliadin portion of gluten results in the gliadin triggering an immune response that damages the intestinal mucosa— also called celiac sprue, gluten-sensitive enteropathy, nontropical sprue, and sprue.

Chemotherapy The therapeutic use of chemical agents to treat disease.

CHF Congestive heart failure

Cholelithiasis Production of gallstones.

Cirrhosis Widespread disruption of normal liver structure by fibrosis and the formation of regenerative nodules that are caused by various chronic progressive conditions affecting the liver (such as long-term alcohol abuse or hepatitis).

CKD stage 3 A person with Stage 3 chronic kidney disease (CKD) has moderate kidney damage. This stage is broken up into two: a decrease in glomerular filtration rate (GFR) for Stage 3A is 45–59 mL/min and a decrease in GFR for Stage 3B is 30–44 mL/min. As kidney function declines, waste products can build up in the blood, causing a condition known as "uremia." In Stage 3, a person is more likely to

135

develop complications of kidney disease, such as high blood pressure, anemia (a shortage of red blood cells), and/or early bone disease.

Colitis Inflammation of the colon.

Common Bile Duct The duct formed by the union of the hepatic and cystic ducts and opening into the duodenum.

COPD Chronic obstructive pulmonary disease

CVA Cerebrovascular accident

D

Diuresis The act of affecting diuresis.

DKA Diabetic ketoacidosis is a dangerous complication of diabetes mellitus in which the chemical balance of the body becomes far too acidic.

Duragesic A skin patch containing fentanyl, an opioid pain medication.

Dysphagia Difficulty in swallowing.

Dyspnea Difficult or labored breathing, shortness of breath.

Dysrhythmia Disturbance of rhythm, such as of brain waves or the heartbeat.

E

Electroconvulsive therapy A medical treatment for severe mental illness in which a small, carefully controlled amount of electricity is introduced into the brain. It is used to treat a variety of psychiatric disorders, including severe depression.

Endoscopy An illuminated, usually fiber-optic flexible or rigid tubular, instrument for visualizing the interior of a hollow organ or part (such as the bladder or esophagus) for diagnostic or therapeutic purposes that typically has one or more channels to enable passage of instruments (such as forceps or scissors).

End-stage renal disease The final stage of kidney failure (as that resulting from diabetes, chronic hypertension, or glomerulonephritis), which is marked by irreversible loss of renal function— also called end-stage kidney disease, end-stage kidney failure, and end-stage renal failure.

ETOH An acronym for ethyl alcohol. Ethyl alcohol is also referred to as ethanol. Ethyl alcohol is the type of alcohol found in all alcoholic beverages.

Exacerbation To make more violent or severe. Marked by greater intensity in the signs and symptoms of the patient being treated.

F

Fistula An abnormal passage that leads from an abscess, hollow organ, or part to the body surface or from one hollow organ to another.

Flaccid Not firm or stiff.

Fluid retention A failure to excrete excess fluid from the body. Causes may include renal, cardiovascular, or metabolic disorders. In uncomplicated cases, the condition can sometimes be corrected with diuretics and a low-salt diet.

G

Gallstones A calculus (as of cholesterol) formed in the gallbladder or biliary passages.

GERD Gastroesophageal reflux disease; it is a digestive disorder that affects the lower esophageal sphincter (LES).

GFR Glomerular filtration rate

Glimepiride A drug that functions chiefly in stimulating the release of insulin from pancreatic beta cells and is taken orally in the treatment of type 2 diabetes.

Gluten-free A diet or food that does not contain gluten. Gluten is a general name for the proteins found in wheat (wheatberries, durum, emmer, semolina, spelt, farina, farro, graham, KAMUT® khorasan wheat, and einkorn), rye, barley and triticale.

Guaiac A test that looks for hidden (occult) blood in a stool sample.

H

Hemodialysis A treatment for kidney failure that uses a machine to filter blood outside of the body.

Hospice A program designed to provide palliative care and support to the terminally ill in a home or homelike setting.

HTN Hypertension

Humalog A type of fast-acting insulin.

Hypercholesterolemia The presence of excess cholesterol in the blood.

Hyperlipidemia Benign prostatic hyperplasia, benign prostatic hypertrophy.

Hyperparathyroidism The presence of excess parathyroid hormone in the body, resulting in disturbance of calcium metabolism with increase in serum calcium and decrease in inorganic phosphorus, loss of calcium from bone, and renal damage with frequent kidney-stone formation.

Hypokalemia A deficiency of potassium in the blood.

Hypotensive Low blood pressure.

Hypoxia A deficiency of oxygen reaching the tissues of the body.

I

Ileus Functional obstruction of the gastrointestinal tract and especially the small intestine that is marked by the absence of peristalsis; is usually accompanied by abdominal pain, bloating, and sometimes nausea and vomiting; and typically occurs following abdominal surgery.

IM Insulin Insulin that is injected intramuscularly.

Infiltrated To pass into or through (a substance) by filtering or permeating.

Inhalations The drawing of an aerosolized drug into the lungs with the breath.

L

Levothyroxine The levorotatory isomer of thyroxine, which is administered in the form of its sodium salt in the treatment of hypothyroidism.

Lipase A pancreatic enzyme that catalyzes the breakdown of fats and lipoproteins, usually into fatty acids and glycerol.

Lithium A psychotropic drug used to treat acute manic attacks; it is often given on a maintenance basis to prevent the recurrence of manic-depressive episodes.

M

Metoprolol A beta blocker used to treat hypertension, angina pectoris, and congestive heart failure. It is marketed under the trademarks Lopressor and Toprol.

Mirtazapine An antidepressant drug taken orally to treat major depressive disorder.

N

Nares The nostrils or the nasal passages.

Neutropenia Leukopenia, in which the decrease in white blood cells is primarily in neutrophils.

Novolog A type of fast-acting insulin.

NPO (nil per os), in Latin means nothing by mouth.

Nutrition Support The provision of enteral or parenteral nutrients for people who cannot get enough nourishment by eating or drinking.

O

Osmolality The concentration of a solution in terms of osmoles of solutes per kilogram of solvent.

Osteoporosis A condition that especially affects older women and is characterized by decrease in bone mass with decreased density and enlargement of bone spaces producing porosity and fragility.

P

Pancreatitis Inflammation of the pancreas.

Paralyzed Partly or wholly incapable of movement.

Phenobarbital Sedative and anticonvulsant.

POLST Physician Orders for Life-Sustaining Treatment.

Prednisone A glucocorticoid that is a dehydrogenated analog of cortisone and is used as an anti-inflammatory agent, an antineoplastic agent, and an immunosuppressant.

R

Renal failure Also known as kidney failure or renal insufficiency, it is a medical condition of impaired kidney function in which the kidneys fail to adequately filter metabolic waste from the blood.

S

Shallow breathing A respiration pattern marked by slow, shallow, generally ineffective inspirations and expirations.

Simvastatin A statin drug that inhibits the synthesis of cholesterol and is used orally to lower high levels of cholesterol in the blood.

SOB Shortness of breath

Spider veins Small, twisted blood vessels that may be red, purple, or blue and are visible through the skin. They appear on the legs or face most often.

T

Tegaderm A transparent waterproof dressing.

Tramadol A synthetic opioid analgesic administered orally to treat moderate-to-severe pain.

U

Ulcer Pressure sores (bed sores) are an injury to the skin and underlying tissue.

Stage 1: These sore are not open wounds. Painful, but no breaks or tears. Skin is red.

Stage 2: The skin breaks open and there is tenderness and pain. Looks like a scrape or a blister.

Stage 3: Sore worsens and extends into the tissue beneath the skin, forming a small crater.

Stage 4: Very deep sore, reaches into muscle and bone and causes extensive damage.

Uric acid A product of the metabolism of protein present in the blood and excreted in the urine.

Urine ketones A medical condition in which ketone bodies are present in the urine as an indication that it is using an alternative source of energy other than glucose.

UTI Urinary Tract Infection

V

Venofer Is an iron replacement product indicated for the treatment of iron deficiency anemia in patients with chronic kidney disease.

W

Wasting The gradual deterioration of an individual, usually with loss of strength and muscle mass; it may be accompanied by loss of appetite, which makes it worse.

Wellbutrin An antidepressant medication used to treat major depressive disorder or seasonal affective disorder.